SCIENCE or MIRACLE?

The Metabolic Glyconutritional Discovery

by George V. Dubouch, Ph.D.
Letter to Doctors by Rayburne W. Goen, M.D.
Differing Models of Health by Marcia Smith, N.D., Ph.D.

This book is not intended to be a total replacement for standard (allopathic) medicine, which has its place in the diagnosis and treatment of disease. Any unusual, persistent, or severe symptoms should be evaluated by a physician. The natural, holistic approach suggested here, although usually safer than pharmaceutical drugs, can affect different people differently, occasionally producing adverse reactions which are sometimes confused with a corrective response. If a condition fails to respond to these supplements, you should consult a licensed health care professional to see about another course of action.

Permissions
c/o George V. Dubouch, Ph.D.
dubouch@aol.com

Published by: InnerLife Foundation
Includes bibliographical references

Library of Congress Control Number 2003099485

ISBN 0-9747947-0-8 Pbk.
1. Health 2. Nutrition 3. Toxicology 4. Science
I. Title

Editing by Stephanie Reed
Computer Graphics by Todd Weston
Cover design and drawings by George V. Dubouch, Ph.D.

Printed in the United States of America

DEDICATION

This book is dedicated to everyone who has been praying for answers to their health problems. I do not want to sell you or your family on why you should take these glyconutrients, but my heart says to tell them: Show them, help them to know there is a better, safer way to overcome pain, sickness and disease. This has become my mission in life!

ACKNOWLEDGMENTS

Several people contributed their precious time to my manuscript. Their comments and input contributed significantly to the final result you hold in your hands. To all of them I am very grateful and honored by their participation. I have listed them in alphabetical order.

Chuck Coker
Jo Cornelius
William Coury, M.D. (M.A.)
Bill Farber, R.H.
Rayburne W. Goen, M.D.
Clinton Howard
Gilbert R. Kaats, Ph.D.
Monte Kline, Ph.D.
Ann Miller
Herman Miller, D.C.
Frank A. Moore, M.D.
Stephanie Reed
Franklin H. Ross, Jr., M.D.
Richard Roseberg, Ph.D.
Elmer Savikko
Marcia Smith, N.D., Ph.D.
Ellen Stroud, R.N.

To those who contributed their personal testimonies, I thank you and I am sure many readers will also appreciate your contribution.

Finally, there are those people who encourage and believe in me; I would be lost without their love and support: my beautiful wife, Margaret, my daughter Michelle and my son Darrin . . . and above all, my Heavenly Father, who is the source of my inspiration.

IMPORTANT NOTICE

The information in this book is meant to be used in conjunction with the guidance of your nutritionally-oriented health care professional. The dietary suggestions described here are neither advice nor prescriptions, but are provided for educational purposes only. It is in no way to be understood as diagnosing, recommending or prescribing treatments of any kind.

The author and publisher are not making claims to prevent, cure, medicate, mitigate, manipulate or sedate. These dietary supplements are designed to improve nutrition rather than to treat disease; however, scientific research has established a connection between nutrition and many disease conditions. Everyone regardless of his/her original state of health can benefit from improved nutrition.

Any product claims made by individuals within the content of this book are based upon his or her personal beliefs and/or experiences after the use of glyconutritional products. This author and publisher disclaim all liability for such claims that may be made. The anecdotal testimonials have not been scientifically verified by the established medical protocol and are not represented as providing a balanced view of the available science. These are the statements of the individuals and not the author. Glyconutritional products are nutritional in nature and are not designed for use in the treatment of disease or to substitute for a doctor's care or for proven therapy.

Should you use the information contained in this book, you are making your own choices and are taking responsibility for any program you adopt for yourself – which, thank God, is your constitutional right. In fact, you are responding to the laws of the United States of America. The Dietary Supplement Health and Education Act of 1994 (DSHEA) calls for all citizens to become knowledgeable with regard to their health and to participate in preventing disease and optimizing their diets to support restoration of good health. Neither the author nor the publisher assumes responsibility for your actions.

ABOUT THE AUTHOR

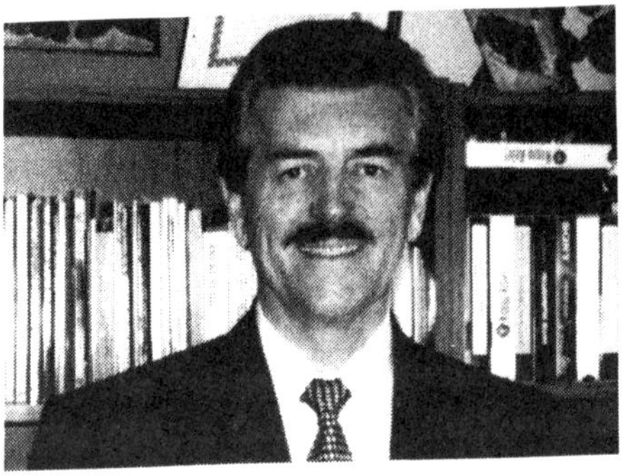

Dr. George Dubouch is a passionate speaker on the metabolic glyconutritional discovery with a B.A. degree in community health and a Master of Science in nutritional science. He lectures at churches, colleges and universities here and overseas. Dr. Dubouch earned his doctorate degree (Ph.D.) in communications from Columbia Pacific University in 1983.

In the mid-1980s he had the privilege of studying under a brilliant doctor, Harold Manner, Ph.D., in the United States and in Mexico. He taught Dr. Dubouch much about metabolic therapy and the immune system. This is one of the memorable quotes from the late Dr. Harold Manner, Chairman of the Department of Biology and Professor of Biology at Loyola University, Chicago, Illinois (1972-1982): "I believe that just as the body tends to reject heart and kidney transplants, so does it reject cancer cells – if the immune system is functioning normally. This process of cancer-cell destruction occurs weekly if necessary." Dr. Dubouch also believes that a healthy immune system will be less likely to reject transplanted hearts and kidneys.

Dr. Dubouch has been around the world exploring diet, nutrients and how to have good health. His understanding about food has taught him, "You are what you eat, digest, assimilate, appropriate and eliminate. If you have a problem with any one of these five areas, you will experience nutritional deficiency and cellular contamination, which are the major reasons why people get sick and diseased." His open-mindedness has led him to study non-invasive modalities and to minister to the total person – body, mind, and spirit.

PREFACE

Over many years our western society has offered us the means to pollute our bodies with chemicals from the air, water, food and industrial toxins in our environment. We are polluted to such an extent that our bodies no longer function properly. We eat too many junk foods and we fill ourselves with health-robbing poisons. We become knotted up with emotional stress from marriage, family, occupation and financial challenges.

Then, we finally get sick. We develop headaches, indigestion, gas, allergies, chronic stiffness of muscles and joints, and a host of other health problems. We are tired all the time and gain weight. Next, we go to the doctor, perhaps have surgery or take additional man-made drugs to cover up our symptoms for the rest of our "natural" – or more correctly – "unnatural" lives.

Metabolic therapy is the use of natural food products to prevent disease and to restore the body by building a healthy immune system. The key to stopping disease lies in an approach that works *with* the body instead of *against* it.

Our Creator has a better plan, a plan for abundant life and health. Since He has made us – body, mind and spirit – we can only experience total health when the physical, mental and spiritual ingredients of health are provided.

– George V. Dubouch, Ph.D.

TABLE OF CONTENTS

GLOSSARY

I placed the glossary in the front of the book so you will familiarize yourself with some of the words and terms that are new and perhaps unfamiliar *before* reading the book. This will hopefully help you to better understand the messages the book is trying to convey.

Antigen: A substance, usually a protein or carbohydrate, capable of stimulating an immune response.

Antioxidant: An agent that inhibits oxidation or reactions promoted by oxygen or peroxides; it prevents rancidity of oils or fats or the deterioration of other materials through oxidative processes. It is especially important in protecting the mitochondria within the cells. Antioxidants block free radicals from causing cell damage.

Bacteria: Small round, spiral, or rod-shaped microorganism that usually multiplies by cell division; bacteria may be aerobic or anaerobic, motile or nonmotile, and free-living, saprophytic parasitic, or pathogenic.

Carbohydrate: A member of a large class of natural substances that are often called saccharides. They are organic compounds composed of carbon, hydrogen and oxygen, including the sugars, starches and celluloses.

Carcinogen: A toxic substance that can alter normal cells, causing the cells to go wild and reproduce at a faster-than-normal rate, increasing the probability of malignant transformation (cancer-causing).

Catalyst: A substance that produces change.

Chemotherapy: Treatment of disease by a chemical compound having a specific bacteriostatic effect against the microorganism involved.

DNA (deoxyribonucleic acid): The double-stranded helical nucleic acid containing deoxyribose found principally in the nuclei and mitochondria of animal and plant cells, usually loosely bound to protein. It is considered to be the autoreproducing component of chromosomes and of many viruses, and the repository of hereditary characteristics.

Enzyme: A protein that acts as a catalyst to induce chemical changes in other substances, itself remaining apparently unchanged by the process.

Epidemic: Disease that affects many people at one time in the same geographic area.

Free radical: A compound with an unpaired electron and no charge. It is unstable and reacts readily with other molecules. They can attach to cells, causing a lot of damage to the mitochondria and DNA and speed up aging.

Gene: A biological unit which transmits hereditary characteristics.

Glutathione: A tripeptide of glutamic acid, cysteine and glycine that is widely distributed in animal and plant tissues. It has a wide variety of roles in the cell for maintaining healthy function.

Glycobiology: The science concerned with the nature and role of carbohydrates (sugars) in biological events.

Glycoform: Molecules, such as proteins or lipids, that have carbohydrates attached to the outer surface of cells as part of the cell membrane. These glycoforms facilitate communication with each other through a sense of touch.

Glyconutrient complex: A standardized new class of supplement in the nutraceutical category consisting of eight monosaccharides, most of which we are not getting from our food chain and diets. Nutrients our bodies need for good health. For more detailed information, go to Appendix A.

Glyconutritional: Carbohydrate dietary nutrient.

Glycoprotein: Any protein containing one or more chains of firmly-bound sugars. These sugar chains modify protein structure, permitting them to participate in functions such as cell-to-cell communication. Most proteins in human plasma and many on cell membranes are glycoproteins.

Glycosylation: The process by which carbohydrates are attached to other molecules to produce glycoforms.

Homeostasis: (1) The state of equilibrium in the body with respect to various functions and to the chemical compositions of the fluids and tissues. (2) The processes through which such bodily equilibrium is maintained.

Hormone: A chemical substance formed in one organ or part of the body and carried in the blood and affecting the function of another organ or body part.

Human interventional, double-blind placebo-controlled clinical trial: In double-blind, placebo-controlled clinical trials, subjects take either the product that is the subject of the investigation or a placebo. This allows for comparison of the product's effects among those people taking the product and those not taking it. "Double-blind" means that neither the doctor responsible for the study nor the subjects taking the product knows who is taking the product and who is taking the placebo. This helps eliminate investigator bias in reporting trial results. In general, double-blind, placebo-controlled clinical trials are the highest standard for interventional studies and provide the strongest evidence for a product's effectiveness.

Immune system: An intricate complex of interrelated cellular, molecular, and genetic components which provides a defense (immune response) against foreign organisms or substances and aberrant (deviating from normal) native cells.

Inorganic: Not derived from animal or vegetable life.

In vitro: Studies done "in glass" (in the test tube or petri dish), usually using specific types of cells that have been isolated from the tissues of living people or animals. These tests give an early indication of effects the product will be expected to have in "whole" animals or humans.

Irradiation: To radiate; diffuse; spread; give out to treat by exposing to x-rays, ultraviolet rays, radium, or some other form of radiant energy.

Malignant: (1) Tending to become worse and cause death. (2) An anaplastic, invasive, or metastatic cancer.

Metabolic: Pertaining to metabolism.

Metabolism: The aggregate of all chemical processes that take place in living organisms, resulting in growth, energy production, waste elimination, and other bodily functions as they relate to the distribution of nutrients in the blood after digestion.

Metastasis: The spread of malignant cells from the primary tumor to other sites in the body.

Mineral: Any homogeneous inorganic material occurring naturally in the earth's crust having a characteristic chemical composition, usually a crystalline structure. Minerals play a vital role in regulating many body functions.

Monosaccharide: A single saccharide molecule, such as glucose, mannose, galactose.

Morbidity: The rate of diseases or proportion of diseased persons in a given locality, nation, etc.

Mortality: (1) Causing or liable to cause death. (2) Subject to death.

Natural killer cells (NK): A lymphocyte that is capable of binding to and killing virus-infected and some tumor cells by releasing cytotoxins.

Neurotransmitter: Any one of numerous chemicals that modify or cause the transmission of nerve impulses between synapses.

Nutraceutical: A relatively new term used by the Food and Nutrition Board of the Institute of Medicine for all natural, standardized, non-toxic dietary supplements designed to optimize health through improved nutrition. Stephen L. DeFelice, M.D., coined the term "nutraceutical" shortly before helping to draft the Dietary Supplement Health and Education Act (DSHEA). Nutraceuticals are also known as "functional foods."

ORAC: Acronym for oxygen radical absorption capacity. This measures the capacity of food substrates, blood plasma and just about any substance in their ability to subdue oxygen-free radicals.

Oxidative stress: A chemical reaction in which oxygen reacts with another substance, resulting in a chemical transformation causing some type of deterioration.

Pandemic: An epidemic over a large region, whole area, country.

Paradigm: A model; an example.

Pathogens: A microorganism capable of producing disease.

Pharmaceutical: Pertaining to drugs.

Photosynthesis: The process by which a plant, under the influence of sunlight, can build up chlorophyll-containing cells, carbohydrates from the carbon dioxide of the atmosphere and from the hydrogen of the water in the soil.

Phytonutrient complex: A standardized formulation of a dozen selected vine-ripened, flash freeze-dried fruits and vegetables designed to protect against free radicals and carcinogens. For more information, go to Appendix A.

Phytosterol complex: A standardized formula mainly designed to naturally support the endocrine system, balancing hormone production with a plant-derived precursor, a dioscorea herb. For more detailed information, go to Appendix A.

Platelet: Small disc in bloodstream used for blood coagulation.

Polysaccharide: A carbohydrate that contains 20 or more monosaccharides. Examples include dextrins, starches, glycogen, cellulose, gums.

Receptor: A chemical structure, usually a glycoprotein, on the cell surface or within the cytoplasm that binds to a specific factor such as a neurotransmitter, antigen, or a hormone.

Refractometer: An optical and precision instrument for testing the sugar concentration for mineral content or percentage of soluble solids.

Substrate: The substance that is acted upon by an enzyme or ferment.

Sugar: As used in this book, a chemistry term often used interchangeably with monosaccharides and carbohydrates.

Therapeutics: Scientific treatment of disease.

Vacuoles: Bubble-like spaces or cavities in the protoplasm of a plant cell, containing nutrients; a place of storage.

Virus: A minute parasitic microorganism that lacks independent metabolism and is not capable of growth or reproduction independently of living cells.

Vitamin: One of a group of approximately 15 organic substances, present in minute amounts in foods, that are essential to normal metabolism. Most vitamins cannot be manufactured by the body and so need to be supplemented.

"Aging should be free from the restrictions of chronic degenerative diseases like cancer, diabetes, arthritis, etc.; our senior years ought to be a time of contribution - *not* a painful crawl toward the grave!"

Chapter 1
THE PROBLEM

You might think you are healthy. You may even have the appearance of health with no pain or symptoms of any kind, but just because you do not feel bad does not mean you are healthy. Disease is a process that sometimes takes years to develop and become manifested to where you experience problems (symptoms). Your body is in a constant struggle to stay healthy. It does not matter where you live or how careful you are in avoiding exposure to toxins and pollutants from the air, water and food. In and underneath your skin is a war zone. Your body is under attack 24 hours a day, 7 days a week, by bacteria, viruses, toxins – antigens of all kinds trying to destroy you. Your body does not care what it is called. What's in a name? It does not even care where it originated, be it a flu, an infection, pneumonia, anthrax, smallpox, SARS, etc. New names are popping up all the time; to your body they are all destructive agents – invaders trying to take over and their effect is to erode the life of every cell with which they come into contact.

Your body knows when it is under attack; it deals with it daily, up to an average of 10,000 hits on every cell in your body by free radicals. It does not matter what the pathogen is, a healthy immune system with sufficient fat-and water-soluble antioxidants will take care of it. But this is where the problem lies. How healthy is *your* immune system and do you have enough antioxidants? If you catch the flu easily or often, if you are run down, if you are under constant stress, you worry a lot, you're in a state of depression, you don't sleep well, you feel weak or high strung (explode easily), then your immune system could be compromised. This is especially true if you have a constantly low level of energy and/or poor endurance. On top of having to deal with contagious diseases, we have chronic degenerative diseases that are not successfully being treated with modern medicine. For example, you have a 50 percent chance of developing heart disease, a 33 percent chance of developing cancer, a 25 percent chance you will develop diabetes, and also a 25 percent chance of developing kidney disease. All of these sub-health conditions accelerate aging.

The most effective defense you can have is to build a healthy immune system using the metabolic glyconutritional discovery. I will elaborate on this in subsequent chapters.

A serious problem affecting a huge population of people is coronary heart disease (CHD), accounting for over six million deaths annually worldwide. When you include strokes and the treatment of cardiovascular disease, the cost is estimated to be $250 billion per year here in America alone. We each have anywhere from 100 to 10,000 cancer cells in our body at any point in time.[1] The only thing keeping those cancer cells from becoming a full-blown, manifested, detectable cancer is a healthy immune system. Did you know that your bloodstream contains hundreds of toxic chemicals and pathogens from the air we breathe, the liquids we drink and the food we eat? Most of these toxins never existed on the planet until after World War II. According to Dr. Steve Nugent, "Today we have over 300 chemical toxins in the tissues of our bodies, none of which were found in any humans before 1940."[2]

The bugs are growing and our bodies are getting weaker; the United States Center for Disease Control (CDC) is already planning for the next pandemic (widely-spread epidemic) flu. The CDC estimates it will take the lives of hundreds of thousands of people in the United States alone. Today the epidemic level of both minor illness and major degenerative diseases in America is alarming. Acne, allergies, headaches, fatigue, depression, constipation, premenstrual syndrome (PMS) and the flu have come to be accepted as normal, unavoidable illnesses . . . but are they?

Chapter 2
I WAS 13 AND WANTED TO KNOW ABOUT CANCER

I remember about 50 years ago when I was only 13. I overheard my father and mother talking about a news story they just heard over the radio. It was memorable for me because of their boisterous reaction. The broadcaster announced that medical science would have a cure for cancer in 25 years. My parents wanted to know why it was going to take so long because they understood that one person out of ten was dying from cancer every year. Their impassioned concern became mine as well, and I asked them, "Can I catch cancer?" They assured me that children do not get cancer (50 years ago this was 99 percent true, and there were no pediatric oncologists). This was reassuring to hear from my parents, but I wanted to know more. I asked how old you had to be to get cancer. (Remember, I was 13 and very impressionable.) My dad said we have never heard of anyone under 35 getting cancer, so don't worry. I thought to myself, wow! That is old! And I ran outside to play.

I forgot about it for many years. Then 25 years came and went and still no cure for cancer. Despite all of the government funding and the countless research dollars that poured into finding a cure, cancer is increasing. Cancer is reaching epidemic levels, going from the eighth biggest killer 25 years ago to the second largest killer today.[3] Here is another tragedy: **The leading cause of death in children who are ages 3 to 15 is cancer.** Is the path of medical care (treatment) we have taken as a nation for the last 50 years working? Or do we need a new paradigm in health care?

Grave's Disease and Leukemia Testimony

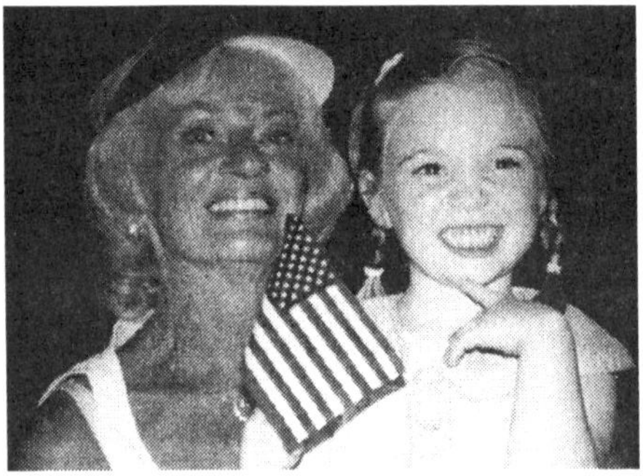

"Hi, Dr. Dubouch. I wanted to write to you and tell you about my personal testimonies with the glyconutritionals you introduced me to. Last September my granddaughter, who had just turned four, was diagnosed with leukemia. Life changed on that day and always will be different. When I heard about the word chemotherapy and read about all the side effects, I wanted to scream; I also wanted to do everything I could to help her get better. I was on trapazole due to a hyperactive thyroid problem and had been on the medication since 1987. Twice the doctor had taken me off the drug and the symptoms came back. I was even on inderal for a rapid heartbeat due to the thyroid problem (Grave's disease).

"After hearing about glyconutrients, I researched them thoroughly, and heard so many testimonials with such positive results that I spoke with my son and daughter-in-law and we were all anxious to try them. I brought all the information to the hospital pharmacy and they couldn't see anything in the products that could be harmful, so her doctor approved all the ingredients and told us that she could take the supplements while she had chemo; but he didn't know how much to give the child. How much broccoli, beans, etc., apples, bananas, etc., do you give a child, was my response. A whole apple for an adult and a fourth of an apple for a child? How many peas for a child – maybe eight – and a cup for an adult? The doctor and the pharmacist couldn't answer my questions and they said they didn't know enough about these glyconutritionals. Doctors *should* know about nutrition in treating their patients, but again, they are in a medicine cabinet and are reluctant to come out because drugs and toxins are all they know. But we were grateful for his openness and his agreeability and we started giving my grandchild the glyconutrient complex and phytonutrient complex in powder form, along with her chemotherapy treatments.

"After just a few weeks, the doctor couldn't believe how her color looked so good and the minimal – and I mean minimal – feeling of nausea and NO hair loss. My granddaughter, Brittany, was taking six different forms of chemo through a mediport which was surgically put in her chest. She was getting injections, IVs, pills by the mouth, etc. One day stands out in my mind so clearly while she was receiving chemo during her hospital stay. While I was there I saw other children around her with no hair, getting nauseous and throwing up. My granddaughter, with all her hair, was hungry and asking for pizza. I'm not trying to minimize her bouts with the hospital or chemotherapy, but I truly believe all her positive responses and minimal side effects are because she is on these glyconutritionals. I can't speak enough about them.

"You probably wonder why I brought up my thyroid problem. While my energy and support were all going toward Brittany, I forgot to take my thyroid medication for four months. This is a pill I had been taking for 15 years to control my thyroid. While my granddaughter was taking the two products, I also was taking these products faithfully every day, and with another supplement for adults called a phytosterol complex. After six months on the products I made time to see my endocrinologist, and I explained that I had forgotten to take my medication. He examined me and took a blood sample. He wrote me out a prescription but told me not to fill it but just to wait and see what the blood sample would reveal. In two days he called me and told me to continue doing whatever I was doing and not to fill out the prescription and he would see me in three months to check it again. I know in my heart I will take these products forever; and not only is my granddaughter on them forever, but the rest of my family is too. I thank God for leading me to these products and I know that one day I will watch my granddaughter dance at her wedding!"

– *Barbara B.*

"If the doctor of today does not become the nutritionist of tomorrow, then the nutritionist of today will become the doctor of tomorrow!"

Chapter 3
THE DISCOVERY OF A GLYCONUTRIENT

What if you could wake up tomorrow mentally alert without pain or health problems of any kind? I have good news! There has been a breakthrough discovery for health and wellness – even anti-aging. I have been utilizing this documented scientific knowledge for over seven years and the results have been amazing! The metabolic glyconutritional discovery has a glyconutrient complex as its basic foundation. It also incorporates other nutrients to facilitate a reversal of the underlying cause of an underactive or overactive immune system, which is cellular contamination and nutritional deficiency.

This is not a new drug; it is not a vitamin, mineral, an herb or a homeopathic. It is a metabolic glyconutritional discovery. Glyconutrients are a different kind of nutrient; *glyco* comes from a Greek word meaning sweetness, so glyconutrient means sugar nutrient. This is not table sugar (sucrose). Sucrose is a disaccharide, a two-sugar molecule; it is sweet to the taste, only used for energy and excessively taxes the pancreas. Consequently, it is unhealthy.

The glyconutrient complex is not sweet like table sugar, and it is imperative that we eat these vitally important nutrients every day. These sugar nutrients even help diabetics by supporting the body in its rebuilding of pancreatic function. <u>Everybody</u> needs these glyconutrients for good health, for healing and to possibly slow down the aging process.

The discovery of glyconutrients and their importance is surprising medical science. Thousands of impressive testimonials, hundreds and hundreds of documented papers and abstracts – even double-blind, placebo-controlled studies – confirm the efficacy and effectiveness of these wonderful, non-toxic all-natural nutritional substrates that rarely, if ever, have negative side effects. At the date of the writing of this book, there are two double-blind, placebo-controlled studies already published on glyconutrients. These studies are considered to be the highest standard for human interventional studies; they provide the strongest evidence for a product's effectiveness.[4,5]

The studies were done through a USDA grant at the Arkansas Children's Nutrition Center at the University of Arkansas in Little Rock. The studies were presented at the Federation Proceedings Experimental Biology Meeting, the largest meeting of scientists in the world.

M.D. News Magazine had a medical update regarding glyconutrition and nutraceuticals called "Glyconutritionals and Nutraceuticals: The Next Phase of Dietary Supplements." It said: "Glyconutrients are, in fact, nothing more than natural food elements that assist the body in preventing or treating diseases . . . Associated with nutraceuticals, glyconutrients are in a class by themselves and constitute a possible important discovery for the health of the body's immune system (www.GlycoScience.org*). This is big news, folks! Don't minimize its importance for health and the economical benefits. The impact of this discovery could be the catalyst for changes in health care as we know it today. **Research indicates nutraceuticals promote the body's self-healing properties.** Dietary supplements are considered nutraceuticals if they are non-toxic micronutrients that are active in cellular metabolism through their support of the synthesis of molecules that conduct innate mechanisms of defense, repair, healing and regulating balance."[6]

* *The World Wide Web honored www.GlycoScience.org for excellence. This award-winning web site is designed to provide information on nutritional products, monosaccharides (carbohydrate molecules) – glyconutritionals – that form the scientific underpinnings for the products and to inform health professionals who are interested in learning more about the safety and effectiveness of nutritional supplementation for their patients. Sections are also written for United States non-health professionals who want to know more about personal choices they can make to affect their health and the health of their families. Finally, for the research scientist, the site assembles in one place, much of the published research concerning the role of nutritional monosaccharides in health. This growing body of knowledge comes from all over the world and spans many scientific disciplines. The site is educational in nature and is not designed for use in product promotion. The information is not intended to substitute for a doctor's care or for proven therapy.*

Over 100 years ago, the creative genius, Thomas A. Edison, the inventor of the electric light, shed another kind of light on the doctors of the future. He said, "The doctor of the future will give no medicine, but will interest his patients in the care of the human frame, in diet and in the cause and prevention of disease." Let me say at this point: **If the doctor of today does not become the nutritionist of tomorrow, then the nutritionist of today will become the doctor of tomorrow.** Look at what Hippocrates, the father of modern medicine, told all of us 2,500 years ago: "**Let your food be your medicine and your medicine be your food.**" You cannot say it any better than that – short and sweet.

Here is more support for a nutritional approach, surprisingly, from the pharmaceutical industry. Paracelsus, the father of pharmacology was once quoted to have said, "**All that man needs for good health and healing is provided by God in nature; the challenge to science is to find it.**" I personally believe we have found a major missing link, a health-building, non-toxic nutrient for all mankind – the glyconutrient complex. Paracelsus Philippus Aureolus, the German physician and alchemist, was born in Switzerland (1493 – 1541) under the name of Theophrastus Bombastus von Hohenheim. Paracelsus has been more recently quoted to have said, "**Everything man needs to sustain health can be found in nature. It is the job of science to find them.**" It is a slight deviation from his original quote, but with a big omission – God has been left out of the quote.

Bill McAnalley, Ph.D., research pharmacologist from Texas, started to investigate monosaccharides at Carrington Labs. Then H. Reg McDaniel, M.D., a pathologist also from Texas, was recruited by Clinton Howard and Dr. McAnalley to work with him on the research team. An unsung hero of early research was Clinton Howard. I would say from what I found out personally from Reg McDaniel, M.D., Clinton Howard started the ball rolling when he raised the money to do legitimate scientific research when there was very little interest in scientifically documenting aloe vera or any natural products. He started a company called Carrington Labs, hired credentialed professionals of which Bill McAnalley, Ph.D., and H. Reg McDaniel, M.D., were part of the team. Research began on the aloe polymannose. "The raising of money," says Reg McDaniel, "to do private research that is out of the mainstream of scientific and medical thought and belief is a real feat." In the late 1980s Dr. McAnalley developed a method to prevent the destruction of the labile principal (mannose 1-4) in this polymannose acetate. This was accomplished when Dr. McAnalley arrested the destructive enzyme present in the compound and then stabilized the functional component. This opened a doorway into a new science around polysaccharides. In lab animal models it was shown that after applying this nutrient, standardized burns healed 20 – 30 percent faster than the leading pharmaceutical agent, with less scarring and infection.[7,8]

In a double-blind, placebo-controlled study conducted on oral ulcers at Baylor College of Dentistry, freeze-dried disks of this nutrient produced immediate relief of pain, and healing was approximately 30 percent faster than those treated in the control group. Multiple reports of scar revision and reversal of sun and age damage were reported. Research continued such that seven additional monosaccharides were identified – and this was just the beginning.

For his work on intracellular communication on how proteins are directed to the correct position in the cell, the 1999 Nobel Prize for Medicine was given to Günter Blobel, M.D., Ph.D.,[9] for his discovery relating to the very science of cellular communication. The last four Nobel prizes from 1999 through 2002 have dealt with the cellular communication process and its importance to our wellness. For proper cell-to-cell communications to occur, it is now believed by many in the know that it takes eight special monosaccharides. These eight essential carbohydrates are elaborated on in the medical textbook *Harper's Biochemistry*, Volume 24, which has been educating health care professionals since 1996 about this glyconutrient complex and its role in health and healing.[10] The textbook is the longest ongoing basic biochemistry textbook used throughout the world for clinical information, the latest case studies and discussions of biochemical diseases. A whole chapter was devoted to the identification of these eight sugars that are needed for cell-to-cell communication.

Of the approximately 200 monosaccharides found in nature (in plants), the eight known that are considered glyconutrients are:

glucose [Glu], galactose [Gal], fucose [Fuc], *N*-acetylglucosamine [GlcNAc], mannose [Man], *N*-acetylgalactosamine [GalNAc], xylose [Xy], *N*-acetylneuraminic acid [NANA]. There now may be two or three additional new monosaccharides, the names of which I am not privileged to know at this time. These eight monosaccharides are converted into glycoforms (glycoproteins and glycolipids) on cell surfaces through a process called glycosylation creating the glycoproteins or glycolipids.[7,10,11] When the glycoforms are present and functioning effectively, it is like turning the lights on inside your body so your defense mechanisms that make up the immune system can see who is friend and who is foe, which cells need help and which cells (bad guys) need to be eliminated. This is an over-simplified explanation for a very important function for maintaining health and life. This process enables proper cellular communication so oxygen, water, vitamins and minerals, antioxidants and other important nutrients can go where needed and metabolic waste and toxins from cells can be eliminated.[10,11]

But it is important to understand that the immune system is one of the most vital systems of the body for maintaining a homeostasis (balanced) condition. Without all the necessary glycoproteins on the cell surface, it is like trying to write a letter to someone without using consonants – it would not be legible. Or, it is like trying to talk to someone without using vowels – the words you speak will not be understandable.

The eight monosaccharides that make up the glyconutrient complex balances and strengthens the immune system like no other product found anywhere in the world. It can up-regulate or down-regulate an immune system, whether it is underactive or overactive, bringing it into a state of balance and optimum health.[7,8,12] With proper cell-to-cell communication, the immune system can be vigilant in its surveillance and elimination of viruses, fungi – killing bacteria, carcinogens and defending against infections.

It is well known that free radical oxygen damage contributes to rapid cellular aging and premature death. It is also known today that when your body has high intracellular levels of glutathione (GSH), the aging process is slowed down. GSH has two major functions for maintaining cellular life and balance: (1) Detoxifying your cells from drugs, toxic chemicals and metabolic waste. (2) Assisting age reversal by acting as an antioxidant to neutralize free radicals, helping to diminish or prevent oxidative stress. Low levels of GSH will put a person at a higher risk for disease, as natural killer cell (NK) function drops. (NK cells are part of your frontline defense system.)[13,14] As we age our GSH level continues to decline, along with a body experiencing cellular contamination and nutritional deficiency. Replenishing our diets with glyconutritional supplements can help maintain high GSH activity and should at least slow down the aging process and build up our immune system defenses.

If you are asking yourself, should I supplement my diet with these glyconutritionals, my answer is an emphatic YES! Everyone on the face of the earth needs these nutrients.

Here is a recent quote from Dr. Rob Ortman, M.D., immunologist and research scientist: **"I believe glyconutrients are going to become a staple nutritional supplement for all six billion people on the face of this earth within the next three to five years."** Here is what another esteemed medical doctor had to say about this scientific discovery: **"The biggest revolutionary change in the war against disease is represented by glyconutritionals."** – Michael Schlachter, M.D., board certified in internal medicine and pulmonary disease clinical instructor. This author believes that one day in the not-too-distant future that metabolic therapy using glyconutrients will become standard-of-care. Today, at age 63, I expect to be alive to welcome that historic moment.

The *Physician's Desk Reference for Nonprescription Drugs and Dietary Supplements* (PDR) is a reference used by most doctors and health care professionals that recommend and utilize complementary and integrative healthcare. This PDR lists glyconutritionals as nutritional therapy for compromised immune systems.[15]

Science magazine, the premier journal for researchers and scientists, dedicated 12 articles in the March 2001 issue to educating the science and medical communities about glyconutrients. In the 42-page special report it stated that carbohydrate compounds currently in clinical trials are aimed at fighting everything from inflammation and tissue rejection to hepatitis and cancer. One of the articles entitled "Saving Lives with Sugars" relates how Hudson Freeze, who heads the glycobiology program at the Burnham Institute in LaJolla, California, discovered that using mannose (just one of the eight essential monosaccharides) has had apparently life-saving results for children with CDG1b (a genetic disease). Freeze and Thorsten Marquardt of the Pediatric Clinic in Münster, Germany, also found a monosaccharide, fucose (another one of the eight essential monosaccharides), that works as a treatment for a disorder affecting the immune system.

Another article in this special report, "Glycosylation and the Immune System," gives rheumatoid arthritis, an autoimmune disease, as one example of the connection of monosaccharides needed with various conditions and the new hope for many other diseased states such as cancer, diabetes and Alzheimer's.[16]

Alzheimer's Testimony

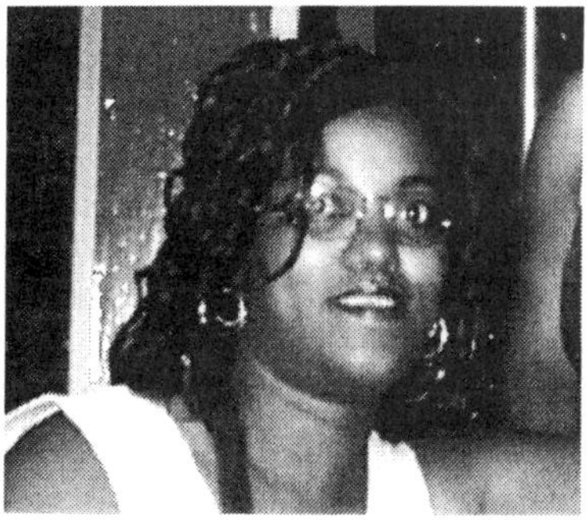

My name is Carolyn and my story is about my mother Annie, a 70-year-old Alzheimer patient. Mom was always a quiet soft-spoken person, but this in no way prepared me to cope with the personality changes the disease caused. She was first diagnosed in 1995 and began taking Alzheimer medicine at that time. Every year I watched her slowly deteriorate. In September, 2002, she had deteriorated to the point of total incontinence, living in a lonely world of her own, not caring who or what was around her and having no interest in anything. She was unable to respond to even the simplest verbal commands. She was losing her hair in clusters and her equilibrium was way off. She needed 24/7 care.

After researching glyconutrients, I began her on the products in October, 2002. I was eager to see progress, so I started her on two teaspoons of the glyconutrient complex every day and quickly increased it to four teaspoons. I also gave her the phytonutrient complex and the phytosterol complex in varied amounts. The first thing I noticed was in four days her hair stopped falling out. Within a week she started opening the door of the car on her own when it was time to get out. This she couldn't do before and hasn't been able to do for two years. Shortly after that, she began to participate in conversations. She looked for a bathroom when she needed to go; she is now off her Depends; Mom started recognizing family members and their names, shocking everyone who knew of her plight. In general, Mother has developed a much healthier disposition.

Currently, with all her health concerns in check, I have gone back to experimenting with the amounts of glyconutritional products. I make sure she has them every day. She still has problems with short-term memory, in that she is never sure what she just did; however, she is always pretty sure of what she wants to do next, i.e., go to the bathroom, get out of the car, tell us she wants chicken instead of fish, things like that. Generally, she is now a very happy, interactive person who never passes up the opportunity to have a good time. Thank you, Lord, we have our mother back!

– Carolyn W.

Scientific American magazine had an article that talked about sweet medicine: "Sugars modify many proteins and fats on cell surfaces and participate in such biological processes as immunity and cell-to-cell communication."[11,17] They also play a positive role in a range of diseases from viral infection to cancer. Millions of dollars in grant money has been awarded by the National Institutes of Health to study how cells and the immune system use these sugars (monosaccharides).

Acta Anatomica, a medical journal, said in its first issue of 1998: "Many of the secrets of glycosciences are only accessible to a closed circle of aficionados, who appear to be the only ones to understand the meaningful words of a sweet language of life . . . its biological significance has long been underestimated. The last decade has witnessed the rapid emergence of the concept of the sugar code of biological information: Indeed, monosaccharides represent an alphabet of biological information . . . but, with unsurpassed coding capacity."[11,18]

If you are a doctor, you might be thinking about these monosaccharides I have been writing about and the fact that a healthy body can make other monosaccharides from just one or two. So, you may be concluding that you don't need to supplement. Yes, the body is supposed to be able to synthesize any missing monosaccharides from the one or two monosaccharides that we *do* get from today's diet and use them to regenerate or manufacture the rest that are essential. The body knows we need all eight monosaccharides to make the glycoforms, the antenna-like membranes on proteins and lipids (fats).

But here is the problem. Our bodies are under constant attack from a toxic environment, a diet deficient in nutrients, a stressful lifestyle generated by the twenty-first century and the aging process itself. Our bodies are having difficulty regenerating new monosaccharides because of at least 15 different enzymatic steps the body goes through in the conversion process. Toxins and other environmental stressors can stop the conversion process altogether. This is time- and energy-consuming for the body, making the steps very error-prone. Since most of these nutrients are missing from our food chain and diet, we need to make sure we are supplementing our diet with glyconutritionals. This is not totally new information regarding the quality of our diet and food supply, as you will read in the next section on "Six Main Reasons for Deficiencies."

Gout and Rheumatoid Arthritis Testimony

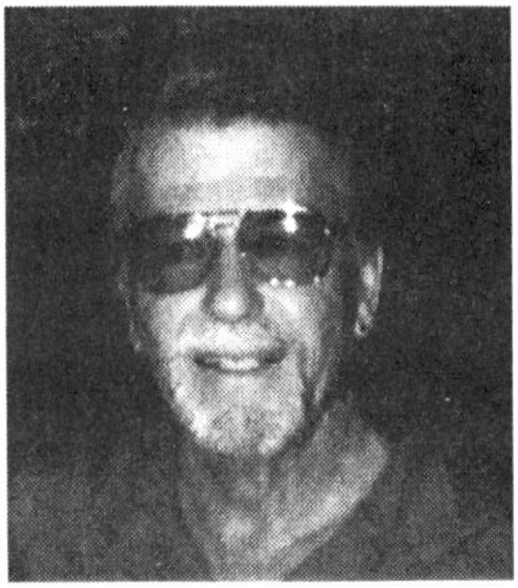

"Five years ago I fell down some stairs and I messed up my back. At the hospital they took some x-rays and found out I had a little bit more wrong. I had gout, tendonitis, rheumatoid arthritis and spinal stenosis in the neck, becoming more and more forgetful; I was a mess. I was forced to retire because it was painful to stand and walk. I was on every kind of pain pill you could find; I just had to take them because the pain was so bad. My brother got me started on glyconutritionals and it just turned my life around completely. They are absolutely fantastic! They brought my immune system to the point where I am able to function like a human being again. I can walk into a store with my wife and not be embarrassed. I used to be bent over, so the only stores I would go into were stores that had carts so I could push the cart and nobody knew I was bent over. I am getting up there in age, but I am feeling great now. I weigh 190 today, which is what I weighed in the Marine Corp . . . lean and mean, as they say in the Marines – well, not so mean any more. Ha, ha! Seriously, I just love the glyconutritionals! They just turned my whole life around and I'll never stop taking them."

– Louis D.

Chapter 4
SIX MAIN REASONS FOR DEFICIENCIES

In 1936 the 74th Congress, Senate Document 264, "Soil Mineral Depletion," had this to say: "Do you know that most of us today are suffering from certain dangerous diet deficiencies which cannot be remedied until the depleted soils, from which our foods come, are brought into proper mineral balance? The alarming fact is that foods such as fruits, vegetables and grains, now being grown on millions of acres of land that no longer contain enough of certain minerals, are starving us, no matter how much we eat of them."

Here are some key reasons why our bodies are seriously deficient:

1. **Green harvest**
2. **Impoverished soil**
3. **Toxic pesticides and chemical fertilizers**
4. **Refining and extensive processing**
5. **Genetically modified foods**
6. **Carbon dioxide (CO_2) levels in our atmosphere have been on a steady rise**

1. The **green harvest** (picking fruit and vegetables before they are ripe) for longer shelf life in the markets is a major reason why our food is deficient in micronutrients. Adelle Davis, in one of her books on nutrition, said, "Eat food that will spoil but eat it before it does." Good advice. Have you ever eaten a homegrown tomato from a garden where the soil was rich in inorganic nutrients and the gardener used no chemical fertilizers or pesticides and you picked the tomato when it was vine-ripened and bright red? Wasn't it juicy and sweet? It was loaded with micronutrients compared to the typical store-bought major chain variety tomato, which is dry and tasteless. Tests done on this latter kind of tomato show very little glyconutrient and phytonutrient content. The tomato was almost void of phytochemicals, which are the natural plant organic chemicals.[19] Nutritionists know that the sweeter the produce, the higher the mineral and glyconutritional content. I have found this to be true using my own refractometer, testing the sugars for mineral content.

2. Crops are grown season after season on the same plot of land in soil that has not been allowed to rest by lying fallow for a season, and crops are not rotated for soil re-mineralization. Our over-intensive farming has contributed to **impoverished soil** in America, which now no longer provides the plants with mineral elements essential to producing healthy plants, which in turn give us the sustenance (building blocks) necessary for life.

An article in *Life Extension* magazine entitled "Vegetables without Vitamins," said the United States Department of Agriculture recognized that a vast amount of our food today does not contain the nutrients it did 50 years ago. Over 100 fruits and vegetables in North America have decreased in nutrient content by an average of 50 percent from 50 years ago. Jane Ramburg wrote an article for the Nutrition Science site (www.GlycoScience.com) called "Canadian Study Reports Significant Losses of Vitamins and Minerals in Many Fruits and Vegetables During the Last 50 Years," August 12, 2002. In the article Ramburg points out the significant mineral losses in fruits and vegetables in Canada and the United Kingdom. This points out the problem is not just here in the United States. The United States Department of Agriculture recommends daily consumption of five to nine servings of fruits and vegetables. A survey published in 1990 reported that only 10 percent of Americans consume those recommended quantities. Now, with the continuing decrease of nutrients in our food, a person needs to eat ten to eighteen servings, although many Americans are closer to a pathetic two servings a day.

Recognizing that standard, conventionally-produced crops are lacking in vitamins and minerals, the American Medical Association (AMA) recently progressed from its longstanding anti-vitamin/mineral position of, "They may harm you," to "They won't do anything except create expensive urine," to now recommending that people supplement their diets with vitamins and minerals.[20,21] This is an encouraging step in the right direction for the AMA. Looking at history, we know that the medical profession will be dragged, kicking and screaming, into the paradigm change of adding nutrients as a treatment protocol. Every major medical advance, from simply washing hands between patients to using limes to treat scurvy, was at first ridiculed, then opposed, before finally being accepted – and then, only when the truth became self-evident.

Dr. Robert Fletcher, and Dr. Kathleen Fairfield, from Harvard University, wrote two articles for the *Journal of the American Medical Association* (JAMA). Their most recent article was published in the June 19, 2002, issue and stated: "Insufficient vitamin intake is apparently a cause of chronic disease."[20,21] This is a big change for the AMA to make, but they still have a long way to go in recognizing the overall benefits of nutrition. Hopefully more changes in this direction are on the way.

3. Toxic pesticides (which include insecticides, herbicides and fungicides) and chemical fertilizers with excessive phosphorus and nitrates all contribute to sick soil which produces sick plants; and when eaten by animals and humans, it produces sick bodies. Introducing friendly insect predators like ladybugs, praying mantis and green lacewings can naturally help irradicate unwanted pests without poisoning the soil. Plants that are naturally antagonistic to insects also help.

In the United States, three federal government agencies regulate pesticides. The Environmental Protection Agency (EPA) approves pesticides for use and sets tolerance levels, while the Food and Drug Administration (FDA) and the U.S. Department of Agriculture (USDA) inspect domestic and imported foods for illegal amounts of residues. The EPA sets the legal limits and they review all old pesticides for reasonable risk. The FDA regulates the licensing of new food additives and monitors all previously accepted substances for harmful effects. The EPA considers 30 percent of insecticides, 60 percent of herbicides and 90 percent of fungicides to be carcinogenic (cancer-causing). It is my understanding that they do not have long-term studies concerning the possible negative effects on human life from specific produce that was highly treated with pesticides and additives. It is obvious to me that food tainted with chemical residues must be harmful to humans.

There are simple precautions that you can take to make your food safer from pesticide residues:

a. Scrubbing the produce under running water helps but does not remove all pesticide residues.
b. Peel the skin, if desired, or discard the outer layer of leaves.
c. Consider buying certified organic foods.
d. Select produce that has no dirt, cuts, insect holes, mold or decay.
e. Eat a variety of foods to reduce your exposure to any one additive or contaminant.

Throughout the years at my clinic I have advocated the importance of keeping energy levels up and how to do that effectively. One day while I was preparing for a talk at church called "Health and Nutrition in Light of the Scriptures," I felt led by the Holy Spirit to Psalms, Chapter 90, Verse 10 (KJV): "The days of our years are threescore years and ten; and if by reason of strength they be fourscore years . . ." (A score is equivalent to 20 years.) There in the Bible jumping out at me were the words telling how to extend life by 10 years simply by raising your energy level and increasing your strength. At my clinic, raising a person's energy level with nutrition was an important aspect in improving their health. It's a type of barometer as to the type of results that the person was getting on the program. The more energy, the greater the ability of the body to cleanse itself. The more energy the body could generate, the healthier the immune system. As also noted in the fifth century, B.C., Hippocrates said, "In nature there is strength." A Harvard Medical School publication entitled *The Green Revolution* stated, "Science fails to respect and retain ancient wisdom." For thousands of years farmers fertilized their soil with organic matter and they produced healthy crops. Shortly after World War II, farming in North America changed radically from natural, organic farming to chemical farming, using pesticides to kill pests, herbicides to kill weeds and economical synthetic chemical fertilizers to increase crop yields. Crop yields increased, but what was not realized by these chemical companies and the farmers using the chemicals was that insects and weeds develop resistance to the chemicals and many of these agricultural toxins were also destroying the life of the soil. Over 15,000 groundwater wells in the United States tested positive for pesticides. A geographical survey released in 1998 revealed that nearly all the streams they studied contained at least one pesticide. To this day, the large commercial farms use poisonous pesticides and toxic additives.

Nowhere else do we see this blatant violation of life carried out more obviously and openly than in the poultry industry. Why are today's hens diseased and dead within two years, if not sold beforehand for food purposes? Why do these young hens produce eggs so abundantly during their first and only year of egg production? The answer on both accounts is that the poor hens are poisoned with drugged feed for greater monetary profits. When you drug an organism, it is being poisoned. Continuous drugging threatens premature death; consequently, the organism prematurely accomplishes a prime life physiological purpose, and that is to reproduce quickly in order that its species may survive. When female chickens are fed antibiotics and hormones via their feed, their bodies react as if they are being poisoned. These salient developments occur:

1. The chicks put on extra weight very quickly, in line with premature development.
2. Reproductive faculties develop prematurely, with a brief burst of intense reproductive effort.
3. The chicken loses vitality, quickly becomes diseased, degenerates and dies an early death.

One of the foremost diseases of chickens is a cancerous liver because the liver is the primary organ of detoxification and bears the brunt of the drug onslaught. With this disease, chickens cannot survive for very long; they are then consigned to the slaughterhouse when their usefulness is over. This happens when the chickens are a young 15 to 20 months of age, or just before cancer is detected. The hormone-drugged or antibiotic-treated chickens start laying eggs at 5 months of age. The naturally grown chickens raised on healthy feed will not start laying eggs until at least 10 to 12 months of age and live at least twice as long as the diseased chickens. So what happens to humans who eat these eggs and chickens?

Is it any wonder why our children are reaching puberty at ages 10 to 13 instead of 15 to 18, as it was 50 years ago? Nutritional deficiency and cellular contamination are the underlying reasons. To develop prematurely is a survival mechanism for the perpetuation of the species. There is an old farmer's saying that helps to illustrate the point: "*Plants that are sickly go to seed quickly.*" When an organism is deficient in nutrients for health and long life, and is subjected to life-threatening circumstances, its survival mechanisms take precedence. This happens in the life of the plant as well as the human body. The procreation process speeds up in the life force of the organism; hence, sick plants go to seed early and children develop prematurely, growing up physically much too soon.

The question for medical science is: "Does eating these types of foods laden with antibiotics and hormones alter DNA programming in our children, shortening their life spans?" The answer to this question should point out the source of the tragedy that is developing evermore ominously amongst us.

4. The devitalization that our food goes through in **refining and extensive processing** further reduces the nutrient value. Let's talk about one example of refining and processing, that of our bread. The white bread that advertises on its cellophane wrapper "fortified or enriched with vitamins and minerals" . . . it's a rip-off, folks. It's like this example. Let's say that you went for a long walk one evening and you are held up at gunpoint and the robber says, "Give me all your money!" Fearful for your life, you hand over all your cash, about a hundred dollars, to the robber and then you beg for five dollars back for taxi fare. In a weak moment, the robber acquiesces and gives you back five dollars; *YOU HAVE JUST BEEN ENRICHED!* You have been given back just a fraction of what was taken away to begin with, and that is an example of what they have done to the bread that has been refined white and has been fortified or enriched with vitamins and minerals. The most recent and most dangerous form of processing is irradiation. Here, food is exposed to extremely high doses of radiation to kill bacteria, parasites and fungi that may cause spoilage. Gamma rays from a source like cobalt-60, in doses of a hundred thousand to three million rads are used. A dose of just ten thousand rads will totally destroy any living tissue. Talk about overkill! This is what is now being done to our fruits, vegetables, flour, nuts, chicken and other foods.

The Health Sciences Institute panelist, Allan Spreen, M.D., in the spring of 2002 made it clear that abundance of nutrients is also eliminated by this irradiation process. He also stated, "Irradiation accelerates the growth of aspergillus mold, which produces the most potent natural carcinogens known to man, called aflatoxins." Processing food with extremely high levels of gamma rays creates some very dangerous molecules.

Nutritionist Jon Barron did an exhaustive profile on the molecular products of irradiation. He points out that the name for the process was originally radiotoxins by Russian researchers. Since that word would be frightening to American consumers, the Federal Drug Administration (FDA) – you know, the organization we trust – came up with a couple of "softer" terms. They call them unique radiolytic and known radiolytic products to describe the molecules that are created, such as formaldehyde and benzene (known carcinogens). The FDA wanted more palatable terms so that irradiated foods would be easier to swallow (no pun intended . . . well, maybe a little intended).

The FDA reviewed more than 400 studies about the irradiation process. They then narrowed their criteria and selected only 69 for in-depth review. Of these, the FDA itself reported that *32 of the 69 showed adverse effects*. But they ended up basing their decision on only five studies. In the FDA's final report approving food radiation, they wrote: "When up to 35 percent of the lab animal diet was radiated, feeding studies had to be terminated because of premature mortality or morbidity."

Look for a symbol called the *radura* which is required on the packaging of irradiated foods. The radura is a green circle (broken into four segments at the top of the circle), enclosing a flower image represented by a large green dot with two petals below the dot. Not all food products will have this symbol, as the FDA only requires the label if, and only if, it was radiated as a whole food, like an orange, which might have the symbol; but orange juice would not. In other words, if you process it in any way, if you add any other ingredients to it, it no longer requires a label stating that it was radiated. As an example of the problem with trusting labels, a product can be labeled organic with only ten percent of its contents actually being organic. This is still misleading and the labels *should* say the percentage, whether it is 10, 50 or 100 percent. This is not an unreasonable request.

Don't think for one moment that just because a food is passed by the FDA that it is safe. For example, there is a strong body of evidence that the sweetening agent aspartame, a neurotoxin, has chemical components which easily transcend the blood-brain barrier and interfere with normal nerve cell function, destroying nerve cell integrity. Aspartame has been linked to case studies causing irritability, dizziness, headaches, weakness, insomnia, memory loss and damage to the optic nerve. Another artificial sweetener, saccharine, is a carcinogen; it has been proven to cause cancer in laboratory animals. You can see documentation of this already on food labeling on store shelves. This should convince you to stop or never use any artificial sweetener. Know that aspartame negatively affects your glutathione (GSH), and the methanol component in it breaks down into formaldehyde-formic acid components which denaturize and mutate your DNA, eventually negatively affecting organ systems. Aspartame was passed by the FDA as a safe food additive. Shortly after it was passed, FDA Commissioner Arthur Hall Hayes resigned and went to work for G. D. Searle Laboratory, the company that manufactures aspartame. You draw your own conclusion. Aspartame is sold as Nutrasweet, Equal, Spoonful, Canderel, Benevia; and it is in thousands of foods and diet drinks. This food additive should be outlawed for human consumption, and just kept as a rat killer, where it belongs, and not in our food and drinks.

5. The American Institute for Cancer Research says the verdict is still out on **genetically modified foods (GE)**. Why then, were 100 million acres of genetically modified food crops planted in the year 2002? In Iowa, corn farmers planted one percent of their crop with genetically engineered (GE) Starlink seed which is not approved for human consumption. Within 12 months, 50 percent of the entire Iowa corn crop tested positive for traces of the Starlink gene. Is the science of genetic engineering of our food proven to be safe? I am not saying my mind is made up – don't confuse me with the facts. I am just waiting for the facts before making up my mind whether or not to jump on the genetic bandwagon; from what

I know right now, I'm not going to. I am not a genetic engineer, so forgive me for questioning; but what about the fact that when you crossbreed a mare and a donkey, the offspring is a mule that cannot reproduce? While this is not a plant, I want to know the pros and cons about plant genetic engineering before I can make an educated decision to support or repel the activity. What happens when these plants are released into our ecosystem? David Gould of Farm Verified Organic in *Scientific American*, reported that GE canola (corn) containing an herbicide-resistant gene, has spawned super weeds in Canada that are resistant to known herbicides. Genetic pollution from pollen drift is spreading throughout North America's farmland. Scientists have been altering the genetic makeup with the tools of biotechnology by inserting a gene directly into a plant to give it a new characteristic. I say, don't fool with Mother Nature – the adverse effects could be devastating. At least, don't jump the gun just because it is profitable. Think about our future generations.

Please, we need long-term human safety tests to be conducted on the consumption of genetically engineered foods. There should be a moratorium on the planting of GE crops, pending environmental and human safety studies. All the foods containing GE ingredients should be labeled as such. Genetic engineering our food or radiating it . . . it all contributes to the devitalization and the derangement of the few remaining nutrients. Recently, the United Nation's Food and Health Organization reported that "organically produced foods have lower levels of pesticide and veterinary drug residues and, in many cases, lower nitrate contents . . . in addition, the 'organic' label provides assurance to consumers that no food ingredient has been subject to irradiation and that GMOs (genetically modified organism) have been excluded." My suggestion is to buy and eat certified organic foods for the reasons just mentioned and because they have more nutrients and taste better. To make the claim that the food produced is "certified organic," the processors' facilities are inspected and certified annually to ensure compliance with all organic standards. The processors are required to maintain a complete paper trail from the farm to the facilities, proving that all ingredients come from organic sources.

6. Here is a little-known fact people around the world are not aware of as yet, a problem of major significance which negatively impacts the nutritional value of plants worldwide. **Carbon dioxide (CO_2) levels in our atmosphere have been on a steady rise**; they are now up to 30 percent higher than they were about a hundred years ago. If they continue to climb at the present rate, they will double the current levels in the next hundred years to approximately 550 parts per million.

Princeton biologist Irakli Loladze wrote in an article ("Plague of Plenty") in the *New Scientist* publication, November 30, 2002: "We may have overlooked a potentially devastating consequence of rising CO_2 levels. It might be a boon to plants, but higher levels of the gas could trigger a pandemic of human malnutrition." CO_2 does promote plant growth, and big agricultural farmers like the idea of larger crop yields and faster growing plants which will make food more plentiful. This all sounds good on the surface, but Loladze believes we should be deeply concerned about the quality of the food we are growing in this higher CO_2 level. Crops grown in an atmosphere of elevated CO_2 are nutritionally barren of micronutrients, particularly vitamin A, iron and zinc.

The plants' nutritional elements mostly come from the soil, converting inorganic nutrients to organic. Photosynthesis captures electromagnetic energy from the sun, with H_2O and CO_2 from the atmosphere, and transforms it into carbohydrates and many important monosaccharides. This 30 percent higher level of CO_2 is increasing photosynthesis. According to Peter Curtis of Ohio State University, when more abundant CO_2 ramps up photosynthesis, plants make more carbohydrate than they can use to grow and fuel their metabolism. They respond by stuffing this spare starch and sugar into their vacuoles (huge cellular storage depots for water and nutrients) so the plant ends up with higher than normal levels of carbohydrate, which means the relative levels of other important nutrients fall (see the 1936 paper referenced at the beginning of this chapter). On top of this phenomenon, excess CO_2 stifles the plant's ability to absorb nutrients from its root system and its leaves. For the world to have healthier plants, the levels of CO_2 should be at or below 285 parts per million; today's level is well over 300.

Rising CO_2 is not the only atmospheric change infected by human activity. Ozone levels are also on the upswing as well as ultraviolet light and temperatures. All of these elevated levels will affect plant health. Loladze says intervention will come. My concern is what kind of intervention? He said, "To avoid malnutrition you have to consume more calories. To keep the same calorie intake, you have to accept a diet low in essential elements. In either case, not a healthy choice."

My guess regarding intervention, which is not my choice, will be biofortification to boost micronutrient levels through genetic engineering. I think this will compound the problem years down the road. Who will be in favor of this methodology? The big agricultural farmers – that's who, because they are driven primarily by yield, not the quality of nutrient content in the produce. There is no incentive for these farmers to keep plant composition optimal for humans. ***Wake up, world, and start sniffing the produce – not just smelling the roses!***

The above discussion points to some of the reasons why we are the most overfed and undernourished people in the world. Undernourishment is generally regarded worldwide as the most frequent cause of immune deficiency and may be a contributing reason for obesity. Throughout history, malnutrition caused by famine has preceded plagues. Today our Standard American Diet (SAD) or our Modern American Diet (MAD), whichever the diet is called, is greatly responsible for our depressed or overactive immune systems. As mentioned earlier, the two main areas that negatively affect our immune systems are nutritional deficiency and cellular contamination. If you have one problem, you will also develop the other. Could this be the reason our immune systems have decreased in the percentage of effectiveness by 25 percent from just two decades ago? And our immune systems are still dropping just under three percent, on average, per person per year![18]

Chronic Fatigue and Fibromyalgia Testimony

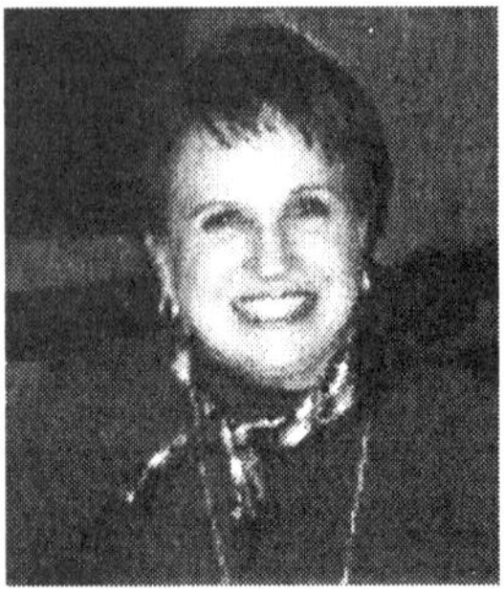

"I have been a registered nurse for a number of years and have been a health consultant, and I thought I was doing everything right – by the book. An apple a day is supposed to keep the doctor away. It turns out that there is perhaps a little more that we have to think about in this day and age with all the toxins and things in our environment. In 1994 I was unfortunate enough to be diagnosed with chronic fatigue syndrome as well as fibromyalgia. Sometimes people have a mild version of it, but unfortunately for me, every organ system in my body was negatively affected such that at the worst of it I would take four hours to recover from walking up just 10 to 12 steps and on the return, it would take me about an hour to recover when I came down the stairs. In addition, I had what I call 'fuzzy brain syndrome' (brain fog where you can't really tell what you are doing) and all kinds of hormone-related things – hot flashes, night sweats, and then of course the aching and muscle stiffness. It felt like I was pushing pre-formed cement around. In other words, I didn't want to sit for too long because maybe I wouldn't get up. That was the picture of me in 1994. And life was basically over unless something major changed.

"I see in the Bible it doesn't say much about prescription drugs. I felt like there must be an answer from our diet and nutrition. I got some help from a naturopath initially for a few months and was making some slow progress; but it was very expensive in terms of the number of things she was having me take. Then somebody introduced me to a research and development company that said they had some research behind the things they were offering. I was a little skeptical but I did some investigating because of my medical background, and it looked to me like what it was going to do was plug some basic holes that we all have because we aren't getting enough of what we should from the food we have to eat.

"So, lo and behold, just within a few short weeks of taking a combination of things like the glyconutrient complex, the phytonutrient complex (key ingredients from fruits and vegetables) and something to improve and help bolster the adrenal system, a phytosterol complex, it felt like the lights turned on – lights, camera and action – and I started seeing my symptoms melt away, just like butter . . . like fading into the background. Probably within about two months all of the major symptoms were basically gone and I had my life back from that time on, and it has been almost seven or eight years now. Not only have I had my life back, but I got excited because this was a major gap that we weren't addressing very well with our traditional medical approach here in this country. I started telling everybody else about it because I wanted them to feel as good as I did. I am happy to report that with a large number of people I have seen their bodies respond very similarly to mine. If you give yourself the right kinds of nutrients and plug the nutritional gaps, the lights go on – healing, restoration and repair are truly possible. I am very happy about that."

– *Ellen S., R.N.*

“Wake up world and start sniffing the produce - not just smelling the roses!”

Chapter 5
HUNZAKUTS LIVE TO 120 YEARS OLD

Here is a true and interesting story I think you will enjoy. After the fall of Alexander the Great, some of the Greek soldiers went AWOL. They escaped from the army near Pakistan and went up the Hunza River when it was frozen. By springtime, the ice melted and no one could follow them. This took place 2,300 years ago. Today, the Hunza people, called Hunzakuts, are made up of three groups: Greeks, Iranians and Mongols.

In the early 1920s, the Surgeon General of England heard stories about a people living in the land of Hunza in the Kara-Koram range in Kashmir, living inordinately long and healthy lives. He heard that they were free of most of the diseases that affected the rest of the world. Their teeth, hearing and eyesight remained good well into their senior years – nineties and up. Their energy levels stayed high also, and it was not unusual for the people to reach 120 years of age. These were the Hunzakuts, who hundreds of years earlier fled tyranny and persecution to hide in peace in the Himalayan Mountains.

Due to the limited amount of land available for grazing livestock, gardens were their only option for food, with the occasional fish from mountain lakes and streams and wild fowl caught from the lower elevations. To increase gardening space, the Hunzakuts terraced the mountainsides. They took very good care of their soil, using natural fertilizers, composting and rotating crops – everything to enrich the soil.

Shortly after hearing about these stories, the Surgeon General of England went to the Hunza land to see for himself and to study the people, hoping to bring back to England all the good news about their secrets for their longer and healthier lives. He stayed there analyzing their diet and general lifestyle for seven years. One day he came to the realization that their overall lifestyle was basically simple but robust . . . nothing that could not be accomplished elsewhere in the world. He noticed their diet was simple, the food unrefined; they did not overeat and their pace of life had very little stress. Their special attention and care of their garden soil and the crops they produced were an eye-opener.

Just before leaving the Hunza land, he conducted a unique experiment, taking soil from the Hunza gardens down the mountains, across the Hunza River to the flatlands where the people raised livestock. These people did not take the same meticulous care of their garden soil, and they did not have the kind of long life and quality of health the Hunza people enjoyed. The Surgeon General built raised beds using soil from both areas, alternating rows of Hunza dirt with rows of flatland dirt, creating several rows. He then planted different fruit and vegetable seeds and made sure the garden was watered evenly. All the rows got seeds from the same batch, the same amount of water and, of course, sunlight.

The results were obvious: every other row had plants that were bigger with more produce. They were lush in color, visually appealing, and the produce was sweet and juicy. This did not surprise the Surgeon General, as he had been eating identical produce up in the mountains for quite awhile. What did surprise him from this experiment was to have a lasting impression; it gave him the answers he was looking for on how to have good health and long life. Reading about his discovery had an impact on my life as well. What he witnessed in the garden was an infestation of insects attacking every other row of plants. Can you guess which row the insects were attacking? If you picked the juicier, sweeter, better-tasting fruits and vegetables, you are wrong. The insects were devouring the weaker, tasteless produce. The question to ask is, why?

I believe our God created insects to consume the food that is not fit for the temple (human bodies) He created. The inferior produce lacked important nutrients and especially antioxidants because of the devitalized soil it was grown in. Isn't it interesting how man, in his arrogant wisdom, created pesticides to kill the insects that eat the inferior food? Quantity, not quality, has been the order of the day. The bottom line has been the money, not the health of the consumer. The Surgeon General's experiment teaches us that healthy bodies come from healthy plants, which come from healthy soil.

Asthma and Bronchitis/Pneumonia Testimony

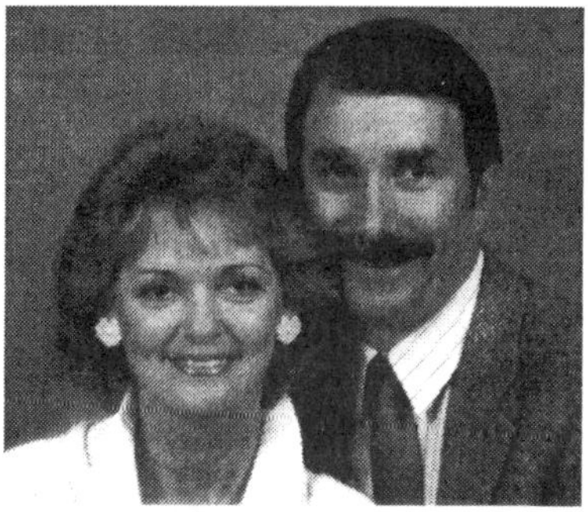

"My wife and I started taking these glyconutritional products about five years ago; and at the time that we were introduced to them, my wife suffered severe asthma conditions throughout the fall and winter of every year. The doctors had given up on what to do for her. She couldn't take any more of the potent medicine that she was supposed to take, so we both began to take these products. She gradually improved – it probably took about two or three years but very seldom does she have to take anything for her asthma. She goes almost the whole year free of asthma attacks.

"I have seen a lot of improvement in myself. I used to get bronchitis. I would get a cold every October/November that I couldn't get rid of, and by January I would be into a condition where I would have to go to the doctor. He would always tell me I had bronchitis or bronchitis/pneumonia. Since taking the products, that has disappeared completely. Those are things that are very noticeable, but the thing that other people noticed about our lives was the overall improvement of health. We praise the Lord for our being introduced to these products because it gives us a higher quality of life; and as such, other people notice that and ask the question: What are you doing different? And we have the opportunity to share the gift with them also."

– Pastor Bill H.

"I believe that our Creator designed us to leave this life quietly, with dignity at a ripe old age without immense pain and long suffering - a change that comes silently in our sleep."

Chapter 6
A NEW LAW HELPS PEOPLE BECOME INFORMED

Dr. Beverly Winikoff, who was with the Rockefeller Foundation in New York, said this in a press conference on January 14, 1977, in the Dirksen Senate Office Building: "Appropriate public education must emphasize the unfortunate but clear limitations of current medical practice in curing the common killing diseases. Once hypertension, diabetes and arteriosclerosis of heart disease are manifest, there is in reality very little that medical science can do to return a patient to normal physiological function. As awareness of this limitation increases, the importance of prevention will become all the more obvious."

On the same day in the same location, Dr. Philip Lee, Professor of Social Medicine and Director of the Health Policy Program, University of California, San Francisco, made this statement: "As a nation we have come to believe that medicine and medical technology can solve our major health problems. The role of such important factors as diet in cancer and heart disease has long been obscured by the emphasis on the conquest of these diseases through the miracles of modern medicine. **Treatment, not prevention, has been the order of the day. The problem can never be solved merely by more and more medical care.**"

We can put a man on the moon, clone an animal; but we cannot seem to change the fact that we are getting degenerative diseases like cardiovascular and osteoarthritis at younger and younger ages. Today, a majority of the people over 27 years old have some signs of these old persons' conditions. Heart disease, hypertension, cancer and diabetes are the major diseases that kill us today; they are epidemic in our population.

Stroke, Diabetes and Overweight Testimony

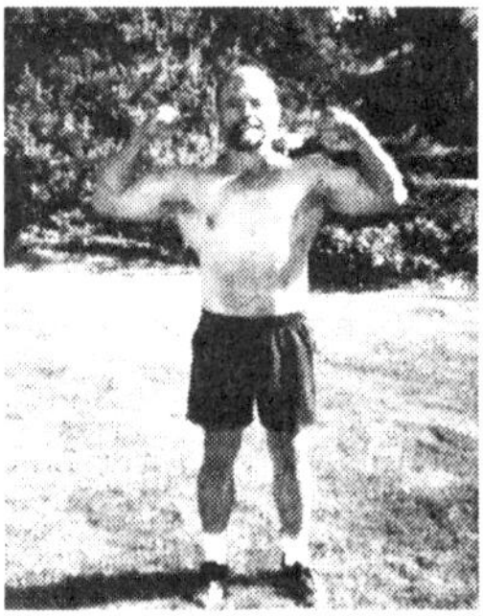

Hello! I'm Michael. Today I'm a happy and healthy person. This wasn't the case six years ago when I was 47. At that time I had a stroke and two years later had a double bypass. I then was diagnosed with adult onset diabetes (Type II) and weighed 246 lbs. and I'm 5 ft. 10 in.; I was tired all the time, my thinking was fuzzy and to top it all, my blood pressure was off the scale. My doctor had me on six different prescription drugs. According to my doc, I was a prime candidate to die. I was not a happy camper.

To make a long story short, two and a half years ago my son, Matthew, a health and fitness trainer, helped me turn my life, or lack of it, around. He taught me how to eat right and to work out properly and he kept pushing me to stay with it, which was a biggie for me. He brought glyconutritionals into my life. It was like night and day – what it did for me. Now if you want to see me, you will have to work hard to catch me. I'm trim and have never been stronger in my whole life than I am right now. I lost quite a few inches and over 50 lbs. I'm on a roll these days and my life is great! I'm alive, my mind is clear for the first time in years, I have more energy than anyone can believe and life is wonderful. I am so thankful for my second chance in life and I am sharing my new excitement for life with everyone. These glyconutritionals put me over the top. It's a great view from here! Come and join Matt and I. I thank God for my son and what he did for me. I am truly blessed.

– Michael H.

In a recent law passed by the United States Congress, it stated, "Consumers should be empowered to make choices about preventative health care programs based on data from scientific studies of health benefits related to particular dietary supplements." Without this new law, which was passed in 1994 and is called the Dietary Supplement Health and Education Act (DSHEA), we Americans would not have access to good information that scientifically documents nutrition and this metabolic glyconutritional discovery. DSHEA was passed by Congress in response to demands of a large population of the nation's citizenry. Members of Congress were deluged by their constituents who were interested in having a more direct access to the power of phytochemicals contained in newly formulated dietary supplements due to their benefits in maintaining and restoring health. Doctors and scientists are recognizing these micronutrients that are primarily synthesized from plants. Acknowledging their safety, many doctors consider them essential for optimal human cellular function.

According to an article in the *Grapevine*, "Previous food and drug regulations were inappropriate as they related to this new class of products called nutraceuticals and the existing regulations of the FDA did not provide a means for educating the public of their value. With the passage of DSHEA, Congress established a new law which allows companies to offer their products to consumers and is the basis under which all nutraceutical companies and their marketing representatives must operate." The article goes on and says, "DSHEA was a milestone in the area of consumer education for products regulated by the FDA. Under DSHEA, nutraceutical companies, through their marketing representatives, are now provided an opportunity to educate consumers about the dietary supplements which they manufacture in ways that aren't possible for other FDA-regulated products."[22]

The greatest bulwark against ignorance and the special interest groups that have contributed to a nation of sick people is an informed public. What people eat is affected in part by what scientists know, or by what health care professionals tell them, or even by what they themselves understand to be true. It is also affected by government decisions in the area of economics, agricultural policy, transportation, food processing, marketing, income, as well as food availability and palatability. Consequently, nutrition today is the end result of the pushes and pulls from many directions, positive and negative, creating the national nutritional environment we now have, which is poor and unhealthy.

An informed nation can stop the slippery, sliding downward slope our health has been following over the last 50 years – but only if we, as a people, heed the red-flag warnings of the increasing degenerative diseases and the high cost of health care. Americans, on average, spend $5,000 per household on medical expenses and drugs per year. The economic burden due to the loss of productivity just from a simple cold is about $25 billion annually.[23] Health care futurist and medical product inventor of 27 medical patents, Nicholas J. Webb in his book *The Cost of Being Sick* said: "Lousy nutritional habits, a 'treatment vs. prevention' medical industry mindset, and the high cost of paying for prescription drugs are all merging to create a health care 'perfect storm' that will, if left unattended, swallow the health care industry whole and take a lot of Americans down with it."

Mr. Webb went on to share in his book some startling statistics and predictions. He said, "Medical bills will become a leading cause of personal bankruptcy. Imagine monthly health care bills of more than $1,000 per month, or paying $12,000 per year for health care on a salary of $40,000. That's where we are heading – health care bills will soon rival mortgage bills in terms of dollar volume." On page 6 of his book, Mr. Webb said, "According to a recent study from Fidelity Investments, a couple retiring today at age 65 would need approximately $160,000 in savings to cover their retirement medical expenses, assuming that they do not have an employer-sponsored plan. With health care costs rising anywhere from 7 to 15 percent per year (depending on which study you use), that figure will equal $500,000 to $2,225,000, respectively, in 20 years.

"So if you are 45 years of age and looking to retire at age 65, don't count on any retirement health insurance benefits. Corporate America will have long since passed that responsibility over to you." Here's a prediction Mr. Webb shared at a lecture I attended in Portland, Oregon, on August 30, 2003.

"Much like our current credit scoring system that we have today, Americans will soon be 'rated' by health care insurers on the level of their health – good or bad. Health insurance companies will use health scores to gauge a person's health risk levels." Now you know what this will do for insurance rates individually and collectively for businesses. Health premiums, co-pays and deductibles will continue to go up and up. Today, premiums already outpace inflation. This rating system will eventually be available to employers and banks and can have negative effects in job hunting and loan considerations. On page 93 of Nicolas J. Webb's book, *The Cost of Being Sick* (2003), he has these fast facts:

"According to *The Journal of the American Medical Association* (JAMA) and Dr. Barbara Starfield of the Johns Hopkins School of Hygiene and Public Health, the U.S. Health-care system may contribute to poor health.

"Annual Death Tolls from Medical Error (stemming from doctor error, manner, treatment or therapy):

- 12,000 – unnecessary surgery.
- 7,000 – medication errors in hospitals.
- 20,000 – other errors in hospitals.
- 80,000 – infections in hospitals.
- 106,000 – non-error, negative effects of drugs.

"At 225,000 deaths per year, doctor error constitutes one of the leading causes of death in the United States, said the JAMA article. Some of these deaths are attributable, the JAMA article said, to unnecessary treatment. Their analysis said that between 4 percent and 18 percent of consecutive patients experience negative effects in outpatient interactions, including:

- 116 million extra physician visits.
- 77 million extra prescriptions.
- 17 million emergency department visits.
- 8 million hospitalizations.
- 3 million long-term admissions.
- 199,000 additional deaths.
- $77 billion in extra costs."

The health care industry in America exceeds a trillion dollars and consumes 15 percent of our gross domestic product . . . that's 15 cents of every dollar. Spending on health care (sick care) is set to hit 17.7 percent of U.S. gross domestic product by 2012, up from 14.1 percent in 2001, according to government estimates. We need to educate our fellow Americans about good nutrition and complementary health options or we will continue to eat ourselves and drug ourselves into poor health, premature death and bankrupt this wonderful nation. Employers around the country are adopting wellness programs to reduce insurance rates and absenteeism; healthy employees are more productive and are less accident-prone. Healthy employees are more creative and happier in the workplace. The crunch is on to cut costs. An example is General Electric Company which is starting to charge more to cover large families. Soon, the state teachers' retirement system of Ohio, which pays benefits to more than 100,000 retired teachers and their families, will stop subsidizing the premiums for spouses and other dependents, all because of the rising costs of the current health care industry (sick care industry). It is increasingly obvious that the metabolic glyconutritional knowledge can have a tremendous positive impact on peoples' lives and our economy, *if people will act on it.*

"There are two obstacles to vibrant health and longevity: ignorance and complacency." This World Health Organization's quote agrees with Hosea 4:6, "My people perish for lack of knowledge." Spread the word – it might save a life.

Cancer Testimony

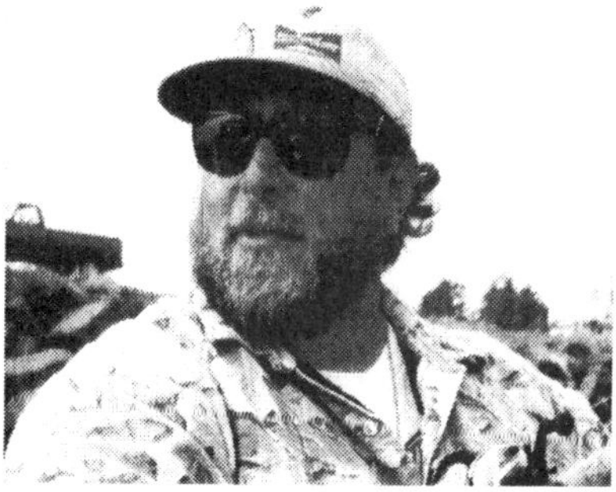

"I was diagnosed with a renal cell carcinoma; I had a cancerous tumor the size of a small football on my kidney. They went in and took my left kidney out and they found more cancer; it had metastasized to my lungs and liver. I was given six months to a year to live. I had met some friends at church who referred me to Dr. Dubouch and to take these glyconutritionals. After three months on these nutritional supplements, my CAT scan came back with smaller spots in my lungs and liver. My oncologist said, "Whatever you are doing, keep doing it." I went on a dose of glyconutritionals that was substantial. After that, my last three CAT scans have come back completely clear. My energy is up and I feel wonderful! So I give the power and the glory to God and for Him putting people like Dr. George Dubouch in my life."

– *Craig S.* (6/18/02) (Alive and doing well: 11/27/03.)

Diabetes and Hypertension Testimony

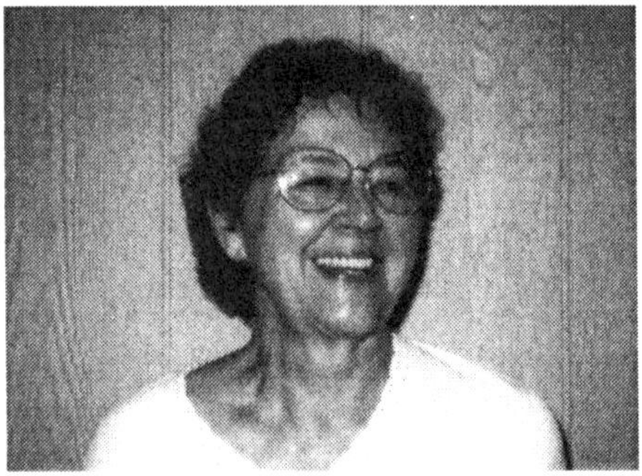

"My first experience with glyconutritionals was after I was diagnosed with diabetes in the winter of 1998. I didn't believe it, but when I went to the eye doctor, he said, "Oh, yes. You have it. You have diabetic retinopathy." Well, that really scared me and I didn't know of any way to get that stopped – nobody does. But in July, my friend Barbara introduced me to the glyconutritionals and by the next eye exam, a year later, there was no trace of retinopathy. At this eye exam there was also no trace of any of the damage that had been caused to the blood vessels after 35 years of hypertension. I think that is a wonderful thing and I want everybody to know about it. My results have encouraged me to stay on the program and I have been able to reduce my blood pressure medicine by 75 percent. I really credit my vigorous good health to the products that I take. I am 78, and I think my health is better than most anybody around here who is this age. I see all my friends in my age group going downhill, as I get better and better. I just hope that God's grace will touch them."

– *Lyola S.*

Chapter 7
THE METABOLIC GLYCONUTRITIONAL DISCOVERY

The metabolic glyconutritional discovery is the use of a glyconutrient complex and other natural food products to build a healthy immune system. It also assists the body's elimination of toxic waste products from pollutants and cellular metabolism. It defends, protects and restores through a combination of immune defense, cellular protection and tissue restoration. It is a multi-faceted program incorporating numerous related elements, each of which definitely plays an important role in the success of the overall Optimal Health Plan (a term coined by Dr. Gil Kaats, founder of the Health and Medical Research Foundation).

Metabolic supplementation using a glyconutrient complex is necessary because without the making of essential glycoforms, particularly the glycoproteins on cell surfaces, one cell cannot communicate with another cell. Through the sense of touch, correct cell-to-cell docking takes place and chemical and electrical messages flow back and forth. Important coded information and translated commands from one cell to the next cell must be quick and clear. This communication linkage is a major part of the body's natural recognition and defense system for maintaining good health and long life.

Immune System Problems Testimony

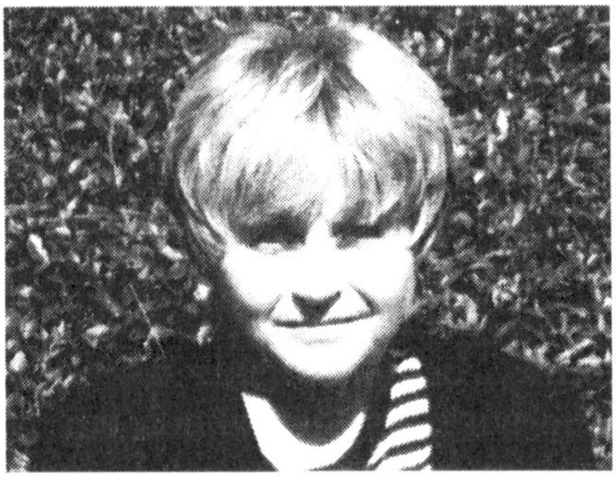

"It was back in the late 1980s when I was diagnosed with fibromyalgia. That was back in the time when the medical profession really didn't know a whole lot about fibromyalgia and didn't do a whole lot for it either, with the exception of writing prescriptions for Prozac . . . and I really didn't want to go that route. I did work with a naturopathic physician for several years. It was costly, but he tried everything. He pumped me full of vitamins and minerals and supplements of all kinds. I remember one day having a huge vial of vitamin B pumped into my arm. Also about that time he diagnosed me with two full pages of food allergies. Now, I know that I wasn't born with a tendency toward food allergies. It was just that my immune system was totally out of whack.

"With the fibromyalgia came pain and sleep deprivation. I tossed and turned so much each night that I would get maybe an hour and a half of sleep. That went on for years on end and I was totally exhausted. I had to take at least an hour's nap every afternoon just to fix my husband's dinner; I was exhausted all the time. I was in chronic pain. Just taking a little walk in my neighborhood would cause my feet to hurt so much that I would be in tears by the time I got back home. I had digestive upsets and a spastic colon. I was also going to a chiropractor two and three times a week. The treatments did give me temporary relief, but they just wouldn't hold. So with all of that, you can imagine that there were many days that not only physically, but emotionally, I just didn't want to get out of bed.

"Praise God, a really good friend introduced me to these glyconutritionals and I got started on the program immediately. I would say that it was within the first three weeks that I saw improvement. I had gone to bed for that traditional hour's afternoon nap and went right to sleep in a nice deep sleep which was very uncharacteristic for me. I woke up a short time later, looked at the clock and saw that I had only been asleep for 20 minutes. Being the great person of faith that I am, I said to myself, "20 minutes – that isn't going to work! Go back to sleep." So I rolled over and tried to go back to sleep . . . and I just couldn't. I got up out of bed and I will never forget this . . . I walked into the kitchen, opened up a cupboard to see what to fix for dinner and ended up cleaning out the whole kitchen cupboard. Believe me, at that time, cleaning cupboards was something I only did when I moved. Well, from there on things just started getting better and better.

"The chiropractic treatments started getting further and further apart. About a couple of months down the road, I was in seeing my doctor and had been bubbling over about the fact that I hadn't felt any colon spasms in quite a long time. His reaction was to reach over, pat me on the knee and say, 'Now, Jeanie, you do know that I hear and see every new product that comes out on the market and I want to tell you, most of them don't work, so I don't want you to get too excited about this. Time is going to tell.' Well, he was right. Time did tell. It was around Thanksgiving, a few months later, when I was back in his office having another treatment. I was chatting about some ailment that I no longer had and he looked at me very seriously and said, 'I can share this with you now, Jeanie. You were one of the most difficult clients that I have ever treated; but today was the easiest adjustment that I have ever given you . . . even your tissue structure has changed.'

"So now it was time for me to get excited. He must have been excited too, because he had another very difficult client who had MS and he wanted me to talk to her right away. I did and she got on the program and is doing really well too. So I guess what it boils down to for me is this. Just as there are too many stars in the sky for me to count, there are that many more miracles of God just waiting to happen. For me these glyconutritionals are a gift from Him and bring really, really big miracles. As you know, my God is a god of restoration and He not only healed my body, He restored my life and I am very grateful."

– Jeanie S.

John Hodgson, in his article in *BIO/TECHNOLOGY* stated, "Almost without exception, whenever two or more living cells interact in a specific way, cell surface carbohydrates will be involved. From the first meeting of sperm and egg, through embryo genesis, development and growth, carbohydrate molecules confer exquisite specificity upon cell-cell interactions."[24]

To maintain a healthy body, cells must talk to each other. There are thousands of different protruding configurations (glycoforms) projecting off cell surface membranes. Glycoproteins unlock the required functions of the adjoining cells and pass on important messages. This is accomplished through a highly sophisticated language of communication where glycoproteins talk by docking with other glycoproteins so chemical and electrical messages can flow from one cell to another cell. This is very important for optimizing immune system defense and to bring the system into a homeostasis (balanced) condition.[10]

For example, when you cut you finger, how does your healing mechanism know what happened? Who tells what systems to take action and to do what to heal the injury? How does one cell communicate to another to bring about the platelets to mesh and mend, stopping the bleeding, healing the tissues? When eating a meal, how does your digestive system know what gastric juices are needed for protein, fat or carbohydrate digestion? Is it guesswork, or is there a higher intelligence at work on our behalf?

The intelligence that constructs a full-grown individual from a fertilized ovum is also the intelligence that heals, defends, repairs and regulates. This God-created intelligence is fully self-sufficient in every living cell. The cell is the fundamental unit of all living things. Its activities constitute what is called the living process. The human body is made up entirely of cells organized into tissues, glands and organs. **The breakdown of the proper functioning of the cell is the basis of disease.** The living cell is in constant motion, undulating and absorbing as well as ejecting. It has a delicate balance. When this balance is upset or interrupted, you eventually experience a response. This response is what we call a symptom or a sign. A symptom is what the patient complains about to their doctor. A doctor in the health disciplines, talks about symptoms and signs. Signs are those things that can be objectively defined by laboratory evaluations like from an MRI or blood chemistry evaluation, etc. There are two ways in which a diagnosis occurs: (1) subjective evaluative, and (2) what can be proven by objective evaluations. Knowing the underlying areas of the body affected can enlighten the healer to know how and where to support the cells and tissues. Realize that each cell is capable of self-governing when supplied appropriately with all the needs for life.

And what a miracle this life is! What transpires within a single cell is staggering to the human imagination. Each cell is like a little city in and of itself, and in a healthy individual, these cells cooperate with their neighbors. No one knows how many cells make up one human being. It has been estimated there are anywhere from 125 to 600 trillion cells that make up the human body. To better grasp the magnitude of a body made of 600 trillion cells, here is a math quiz. If there are six billion people on the face of the earth, and each person represents a single cell in a human body, and it takes a thousand billion to make one trillion, are you ready for some mind-boggling math? How many earth populations does it take to make one individual human consisting of 600 trillion cells?

STYLIZED CELL

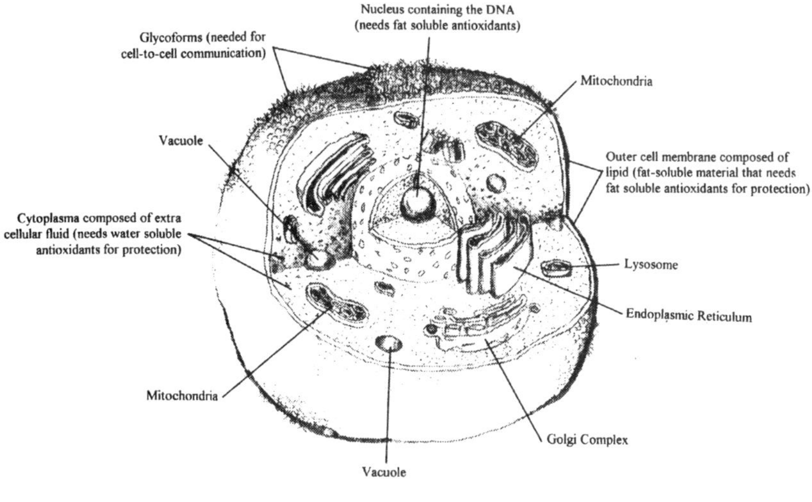

Talk about cooperation! I do not think we can comprehend the magnitude and ramifications of maintaining harmony and accurate communications with just over one hundred thousand times the earth's population. We, as humans, cannot live in harmony on just *one* planet, let alone one hundred thousand earths; but the cells in our bodies must get along if life is to continue. Each cell depends upon the support and cooperation of 599,999,999,999,999 other cells. Let me spell it out for you: Five hundred and ninety-nine trillion, nine hundred and ninety-nine billion, nine hundred and ninety-nine million, nine hundred and ninety-nine thousand, nine hundred and ninety-nine. And all of these cells live together in self-tolerance and cooperation! ABSOLUTELY AMAZING! Even in this maturing age of computers, there is not a computer built today capable of monitoring the activities that go on within just one cell, much less 600 trillion! Is it possible that the universe outside the human body is the same size as the universe within, only miniaturized, and we are the center of the universe or the halfway point from the tiniest atom to the ever-expanding universe? What would be the significance if this was an indisputable fact?

Getting back to the main topic again . . . the immune system is a body-wide network of cells and organs that defend the body against attacks by foreign invaders. At the heart of the immune response is the ability to distinguish between self and non-self. Every cell in the body carries distinctive molecules that distinguish it as "self." Normally, the body's defenses do not attack tissues that carry a "self" marker; immune cells coexist peaceably with other body cells in a state known as self-tolerance, as long as cells can communicate with each other.

If one cell cannot communicate with another cell, or if the messages get garbled, bodily functions break down. The immune system becomes impotent, underactive and disease is the inevitable outcome. The flip side is an overactive immune system that goes haywire and attacks healthy cells and the life-giving glands and organs of the body.

During my research for the writing of this book, I learned that the mitochondria of our cells account for most of the lost water in vital organs (i.e., heart, liver). When the cells' life-giving activities get blocked or interrupted, and especially when they are under attack by free radicals, the by-product of the mitochondria's energy production (water) becomes limited. This reduction in bodily water can contribute to degenerative conditions. Dehydration causes vital organs to become prune-like, the skin wrinkles, and energy levels drop. The whole body weakens and memory and the thinking processes are seriously affected. Dehydration makes you look and feel older than you are chronologically.

Healthy bodies are very efficient in the utilization of water because it is the second most important nutrient to mankind, next to clean air. The importance of water can be measured by the fact that our bodies are made up of about 70 percent water and we can only live for a few days without it. We need water to flush out toxins, morbid tissue and metabolic waste. Water is a main nutrient utilized by our bodies to make new, healthy alpha cells. An alpha cell is a new cell constructed out of new, vibrant nutrients through a continual bodily process of catabolism and anabolism. This is a process of tearing cells down (catabolism) and putting new cells together (anabolism). The process the body uses, utilizing enzymes, keeps parts of the cell that are viable and healthy for regeneration and adds new, healthy nutritional material from food and supplementation. Catabolism is the breaking down and elimination of the material that is weak, old and unhealthy, which we call omega cells. Water is of paramount importance in this overall process of catabolism and anabolism. To stay healthy we need to drink plenty of water every day – pure water, distilled, ozonated, filtered or bottled. Lack of proper hydration is also associated with tissue rigidity, contributing to premature aging.

The mitochondria are like a bacteria within the cell, surprisingly with its own DNA, just like the cell itself. Keeping it healthy is a paramount activity of the immune system. Supporting and protecting the mitochondria is vital in the overall design for life. The mitochondria produces energy in the form of adenosine triphosphate (ATP). After the last of many steps in the process of producing ATP, the mitochondria takes oxygen and hydrogen and creates energy and the by-product is water.

Did you know that 90 percent of our cells' oxygen consumption is utilized by the mitochondria? For many years, I called them "the little fat factories of the muscle." The more muscle, the more fat factories, a key to staying at your optimal size. Well, I now realize that the mitochondria are much more than that. **I believe the health of the mitochondria is key to degenerative disease states, perhaps the underlying cause for all chronic degenerative diseases.**

We humans can go without food for several **weeks** under the guidance of a health care professional and still live. We can go without water for **days** under professional supervision and still continue life. But we can only go without oxygen (air) for a few **minutes**. This is a simple explanation as to the importance of oxygen and water to life, and yet we take breathing and drinking of water for granted. We are a little more cognitive of food. Instead of eating to live, we live to eat – and too frequently, in excess. Could our priorities be in need of readjustment? I enjoy all kinds of foods, especially with good company. I am not a food fanatic; I just enjoy life and try to keep things in proper perspective, balanced and in moderation. It is not what you do all the time that counts, it is what you do most of the time that is important. So, don't stress yourself!

When I realized how much oxygen the mitochondria of our cells use, a light bulb went off in my head. This fact, along with the fact that the by-product of energy production in the mitochondria is water, started me thinking . . . organs shrink, energy levels drop . . . why? Because we are getting old is not an acceptable answer. Every couple of years we have practically all new cells, making up new tissues for glands and organs. Sixty, seventy, eighty, even ninety years of age is not old according to our DNA programming. Our Creator has a timetable for us well past one hundred. We individually cut that timetable short, partly because of the negative things we do consciously or unconsciously, intentionally or unintentionally, to our bodies. The Word says in Genesis 6:3: ". . . yet his days shall be one hundred and twenty years." I do not believe we should be experiencing chronic degenerative diseases at all or at least not until we have reached past the century mark.

As we age, energy levels drop, we become less efficient, our cells' regeneration process is slower and bodily functions start faltering, mainly because of nutritional deficiency and cellular contamination. We can see the manifestation of this premature aging in the elderly, especially in their movements which become restricted. They lose mobility and fluidity in many of their activities. Not only are these signs of aging, but they can also indicate a potential disease problem within the very mitochondria of the cells. When dividing the physiological aspects of the cell into two areas for the protection of the mitochondria, we can see a need for both fat- and water-soluble antioxidants because the cell is made up of both fat- and water-soluble parts (see my stylized cell drawing on page 53). We need to protect the cells. It is important that our bodies have the resources of fat- and water-soluble antioxidants in a high enough quantity to eliminate the free radicals. Clearly, reversing conditions that negatively affect the life processes of the mitochondria could very well slow down the aging process and postpone possible future maladies.

I believe that our Creator designed us to leave this life quietly with dignity at a ripe old age, without immense pain and long suffering – a change that comes silently in our sleep.

How important is it to you to have enough energy in your body to sustain good health and long life? We need energy to fight off invaders, bugs of all kinds, especially the free radicals which attack our cells, as you may recall from Chapter 1, at an average of 10,000 times per day. Energy is needed for all of life's functions; cleansing, digesting, assimilating, all physical activities – even thinking takes energy. About 25 percent of energy production is consumed by our brain's conscious and subconscious activity. Our brains need oxygen and fuel to function properly. The fuel the brain uses is glucose, a monosaccharide from digested food. Digestion takes even more energy than our brain to function – a lot more in some folks, especially heavy eaters of unclean animals (i.e., pork, ham). Meats take longer to digest than fowl and fowl a little longer to digest than fish. Unclean meats, fish and fowl take longer to digest than clean meats, fish and fowl. *This is no condemnation regarding the food you eat; just use common sense in what you eat and how much.* Remember, it is what you do most of the time that counts. Overeating is taxing to your body: more energy is needed to digest and more energy is needed to eliminate the added metabolic waste. Keeping your energy levels up is important to good health and long life.

Studies have suggested that sensible eating can improve and extend life. One such study on diet and life dealt with laboratory fruit flies. In the study, British researchers compared the effects of different calorie-restricted diets on the mortality of fruit flies. They found that fruit flies on restricted diets lived about 90 days, which is twice as long as those fed on a "normal" diet. "The carry-home message from this study," said Linda Partridge of University College, London, England, "is that it is never too late to improve health by switching to sensible eating habits." When food consumption is lower (i.e., calories are restricted) the workload in the organs (stomach, small intestine, large intestine, pancreas, liver and kidneys) that participate in food digestion, absorption and elimination is reduced. These organs then have more energy to be used to enhance life's functions.

The primary biochemical mechanisms created by God are more or less the same in all living cells, whether they are plant or human. The antioxidants that the plants produce to protect themselves, when consumed by humans, become protectors for human cells. Communicating and supplying the right antioxidants and other essential nutrients for healthy cell life is key to the cells' survival. One very important area in this protection process that has been seriously neglected is that of getting enough of the *right* antioxidants. Our cells are not only falling short in communicating needs from one cell to another cell, but our cells are also falling short of proper antioxidant protection from free radical damage.

Free radicals cause oxidative stress, which simply explained is the tearing and pulling apart of healthy cells. Free radicals and their precursors can be ingested and the body's natural processes also create them. The main things that contribute to free radicals and oxidative stress are: emotional stress, pharmaceutical drugs and street drugs, smoking and secondhand smoke, excess alcohol consumption, environmental toxins, food preservatives, poor-quality and over-processed foods, physiological stress and illness. The system disorders associated with oxidative stress include: autoimmune, gastrointestinal, cardio-vascular, neurological and pulmonary – to name a few. Oxidative stress also contributes to premature aging. A recent rat study is showing positive support for high antioxidant diets. The rodents, which have a lifespan of about 2.5 years, are ideal for following the effects of antioxidants on the aging process. A neuroscientist and behavioral psychologist have been testing a variety of foods high in antioxidants. The researchers started the study with six-month-old rats on four different feeding regimens. Three groups were fed various diets with known antioxidant values. The ORAC (see glossary at the beginning of this book) units of antioxidants ranged considerably. The fourth group of rats got a diet that was unfortified with antioxidants, making this the control group.

The study entailed putting the rats through their paces to determine when they begin to falter in memory and motor function. They noted the control group of rats started losing motor function around 1 to 1.3 years of age – about half of their DNA-programmed lifespan. (Note the similarity to human life that this study reveals.) When the rats reached 1.5 years of age (this would be equivalent to a 45- to 50-year-old human), they put the rats through gymnastics, such as walking on thin poles and planks and trying to stay upright on a rotating rod – all tests for motor function. Rodents have great agility and are excellent swimmers, so they had them swim around in a deep pool until, using visual cues, the rats would find a submerged platform on which they could rest. With this test they measured changes in long- and short-term memory. The diets the three antioxidant-fed groups received had better long-term memory than the rats in the control group, which were getting little to nothing in the way of antioxidants in their diets. The group of rats fed on the highest amount of antioxidants did the best. They remembered how to find the hidden platform much better over time, showing that they retained more of their learning ability. What was also evident from this study was how motor functions declined with the control group and how the groups with high antioxidant diets retained both cognitive and motor function over their lifespan.

Aren't we looking at a partial picture of what prevents chronic degenerative diseases? Antioxidants are what our bodies use to protect us against these insidious free radicals. Antioxidant supplementation has been available for a long time and has been recommended universally as a therapeutic agent by almost 100 companies here in the U.S. alone. But the method of testing to validate the content and assay the products' effectiveness in the past has been fundamentally flawed. Previous testing covered only one of the two types of antioxidants – the water soluble. A large percentage of antioxidant supplements available for sale are ineffective or are even pro-oxidants.[25] <u>A new in-vitro testing method now takes into account the activity of not only a single antioxidant, but a combination of antioxidants and not only water soluble but fat soluble and their antioxidant interactions.</u> This testing method ($ORAC_o$) is now the gold standard. High intake of proper antioxidants reduces the risk for cardiovascular disease, cancer and many, many other degenerative diseases. Low intake of antioxidants increases the risks of developing these diseases. The glyconutrient complex offers the highest amount of $ORAC_o$ units (17,254) which can create a significant impact on plasma and tissue antioxidant capacity.

The assayed antioxidants contained in this glyconutrient complex (see Appendix A) is both water and fat soluble. Assembled with co-factors, this unique blend of antioxidants and monosaccharides make this supplement very synergistic in multiplying the antioxidant effectiveness. It has three times more tested antioxidant units than its closest competitor, and on average it has ten times more antioxidant units than most antioxidants available on the market. This supplement has been created to mimic how our Creator assembles plant nutrients which are more bioavailable and easier to assimilate than synthetic nutritional formulations.

Part of your body's defensive arsenal includes many types of white cells. Two types of lymphocytes are cytotoxic T cells and natural killer (NK) cells. To attack, cytotoxic T cells need to recognize a specific antigen (any substance capable of triggering an immune response is an antigen). Both T cells and NK cells contain granules filled with potent chemicals and both types kill on contact. These immune system defensive cells bind to their targets and then deliver bursts of lethal chemicals to kill antigen cells.[26]

STYLIZED

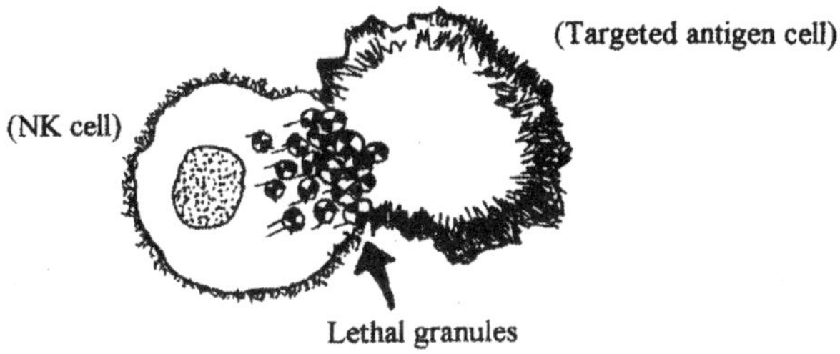

When normal cells turn into cancer cells, the cell surfaces change. These altered surfaces are detected by the immune defenders: cytotoxic T cells, NK cells and macrophages (examples of key defender white blood cells), patrolling throughout the body, seeking out and eliminating cells that undergo malignant transformation. Pathogens and tumors develop when the surveillance system's cell-to-cell communication linkage breaks down or the system is overwhelmed so that the cancer cell is not recognized as being abnormal.[26]

STYLIZED

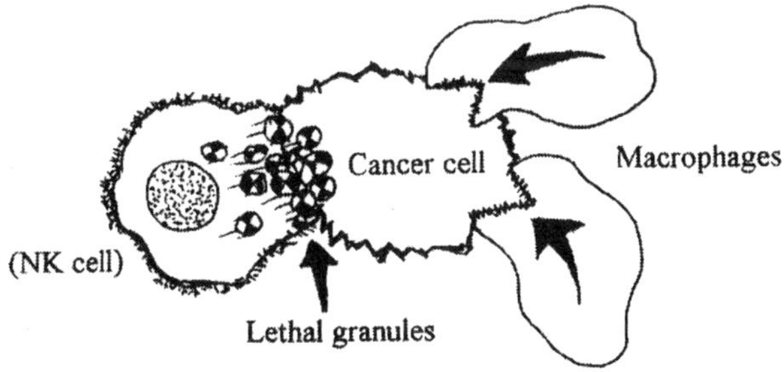

I made this statement in a lecture several years ago at Monash University in Melbourne, Australia:

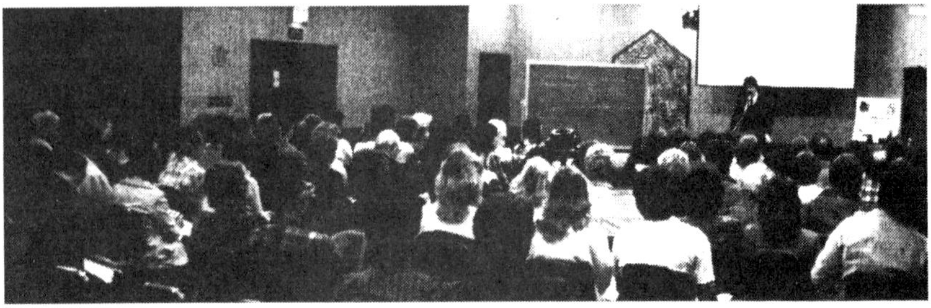

"Your body knows more about what you need and don't need than all the doctors in the world. We just have to stop assaulting it with what harms and start supplying it with what is missing. Then your body will heal itself."

There is no healing apart from God, and no mechanisms for healing exist other than those He created. "We are fearfully and wonderfully made," according to Psalm 139:14. Your body has an innate ability to heal itself. To quote Dr. Roger Williams: "The body heals itself and nutrition provides the resources to accomplish that task."[27] He said, in essence, the concept of treating a disease is replaced by a process of restoring a balance to the body through natural means.

Did you know your heart beats a hundred thousand times a day, your nerves generate three million impulses a second and your stomach produces enough acid to dissolve nails? Every two weeks you have new skin tissue, every six weeks you have new taste buds, and your body is made up of sixty thousand miles of lymphatic system and blood vessels (arteries, veins and capillaries). What an amazing creation we are, and we take it for granted! Shouldn't we listen more closely to what our bodies are telling us? *If you take care of it, it will take care of you.*

Most Americans take better care of the vehicle they drive than the vehicle they walk around in. People live as if they can burn garbage and neglect their physical vehicle, like it was an old beat-up, runabout junker they didn't care about. Then they wonder why they get tired and sick all the time. No one would put diesel fuel into a gas engine, or let their vehicle run low or completely out of oil and water. So, why don't people take better care of their health? Maybe because people remain slaves to the medical therapeutic theory which has neither saved them from degenerative diseases, nor knows what causes them in the first place.

We Americans live in an "instant" society where everything is quick and easy. We have a "quick-fix-it-now" attitude that lends itself to the present drugging mentality which masks symptoms and blocks pain right away, but does nothing to restore healthy cells. Because of impatience and blind trust in their medical doctors, people are willing to avoid asking questions about the consequences of medicines, which all have LD 50 ratings, which means "lethal dose fifty percentile." FDA approval requires that a drug dosage be identified in which 50 percent of the lab animals die from a quantitative amount of that specific drug. This is why all drugs have side effects or adverse reactions sooner or later, because all drugs are ultimately lethal. Have you ever taken, or do you know someone who has taken three or more drugs at a time within a 24-hour period? Did you know there has never been a double-blind, crossover, high-population study done for the side effects for a combination of any three drugs? Yet people blindly accept them without question from their medical doctor.

Voltaire, the French philosopher (1694-1778), said, "The art of medicine consists in amusing the patient while nature cures the disease." Unfortunately, things have not changed that much regarding medical modalities for treating chronic degenerative diseases. The side effects of taking prescribed medication in a hospital setting last year was the fourth leading cause of death in America – right behind heart disease, cancer and diabetes (degenerative diseases). Over a hundred thousand people die yearly from drugs that were *properly* taken.[28] The common aspirin has caused more deaths each year than all the dietary supplements combined. Why do the FDA, AMA and the pharmaceutical industry continue to focus on the symptomatic treatment of diseases with poisons when it has been a diabolical failure in curing chronic degenerative diseases?

I would like to kindly remind the powers that be – the FDA, the pharmaceutical industry and the AMA – about the founding father of modern medicine, Hippocrates, to whom the AMA owes its allegiance, as noted by the Hippocratic Oath (which, to my understanding, is no longer cited at graduations). Surprisingly, what goes around comes around. Hippocrates was the first complementary/integrative doctor (that's right!) – a holistic practitioner, no less! Remember his famous quote, "Let your food be your medicine and your medicine be your food." The words of a true nutritionist. Hippocrates was concerned with the whole body, not just with one organ or part. His concern was with the general body condition; the totality of the sick person. He wrote, "The human body is a circle, of which each part may be esteemed as both the beginning and the end. By the affection of one part the whole body may become affected."

"His chief interest," says the medical historian Erwin H. Ackernercht, "was not for the illness as such, but for the patient. He concerned himself more with the body as a whole than with changes in any individual part." ***Hippocrates knew that diseases were merely symptoms and to treat symptoms did not produce health.*** Instead of treating symptoms with poisons, why not support the body's systems holistically, accepting the fact that the human body is intelligent enough to solve the problems, given the right environment to do so.

I am working with a lady right now who is in her late fifties who has had increasing negative side effects from the ten different pharmaceutical drugs her medical doctor has conscientiously prescribed for her. Since her doctor has become frustrated with the lack of positive results, he was open to the science in the Physician's Desk Reference[15] (PDR) for these glyconutritionals. He became willing to work with me on her behalf to incorporate these specific supplements in a complementary way which enabled her to gradually cut back on her drug regimen.

She said she trusted him and accepted without question his prescriptions for all ten drugs, not knowing what any of the adverse reactions were. Yet, when I first spoke with her about these glyconutritionals and told her that these supplements were made from concentrated nutrients that are missing from our food chain and diets – nutrients our bodies need for health and healing – she just listened. Then I added that this was just food and was not contraindicated to the medication she was taking. After telling her this, I was dumbfounded by her question: "Are they safe?" She is taking poisons and said nothing. I offer wholesome food supplements with proven science and she questions the safety?! We send truckloads of poisons cascading down our throats and permit them to be injected into us simply because we are sold on the idea of "medicine" as a curing substance. In the drugstore, the skull and crossbones are on many containers; but once dispensed, these poisons no longer bear this warning. By some hocus-pocus magic they have now become beneficial medicines. That's the mentality many Americans have because all they're listening to are the voices of those promoting modern drug therapy as the answer to disease!

Wise up America before it's too late!

Weight Loss, Allergies, Hormone Problems, Acid Reflux and Cancer Testimony

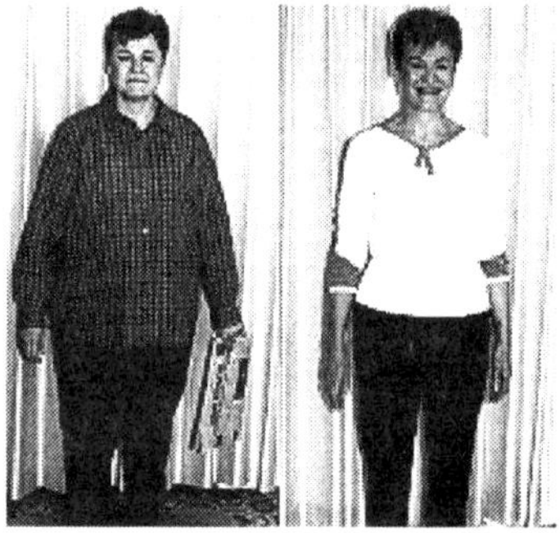

"For over twenty years of my adult life I was a prisoner of my health. I was plagued with allergies, asthma and acne. Then, at age 31, I had a hysterectomy due to endometriosis and subsequently took estrogen to prevent a premature menopause. Seven years later I had a mastectomy due to cancer and was promptly and permanently taken off the estrogen, pushing me into sudden menopause...my hormones were horribly out of balance. The radiation therapy apparently burned my esophagus, resulting in constant acid reflux, even though I eliminated all acid and spicy foods. My bone density had dropped to 81 percent of normal in spite of treatment. So here I was, unable to eat most foods when I developed a severe allergy to dairy products. And then there was all the weight I had gained . . .

"I was a walking pharmacy: 30 years of tetracycline for acne, 20 years of allergy and asthma drugs, 8 years of an acid reducer, 9 years of high amounts of progestin for the night sweats, 6 years of a drug for increasing bone density. My doctors did not expect I would ever be off these drugs, and I finally realized that this would be as good as it would be if I continued on the same path. Then a friend introduced me to these glyconutritionals, and fortunately I was now more open to a new approach.

"Within a few weeks I no longer had hot flashes and actually felt normal for the first time in years. The acid reflux was gone and I could eat the acid and spicy foods again. The acne was under control. Within a few months my allergies were completely gone and I was completely off all medications. This was quite unbelievable! After a couple of years on this program my bone density was at 108 percent of normal and the dairy allergy was gone. I was absolutely amazed at how my body was able to heal itself once I started feeding it these amazing glyconutritionals!

"I was thrilled that my health issues were now history, but I just couldn't seem to get the excess weight off, and in particular, the high body fat. And I knew that being overweight is clearly a health issue. With incredible timing, the same company that developed the glyconutritionals that improved my health so much came out with a new program for weight management. I had to give it a try. I lost 74 lbs. and 36 percentage points of body fat. I ended up smaller than I've ever been! I was shocked to realize that I apparently had always had high body fat, even when not considered overweight. When I last was at my current weight I was two dress sizes bigger. At age 54 I certainly didn't expect to just now be discovering the size I was meant to be! These glyconutritionals have not only given me back my life, but the quality of my life is at a level that I never dreamed was possible! I marvel at how many repairs the body can make when it is provided with all the nutrients it needs. I highly recommend this approach for anyone wishing to improve their quality of living!"

– *Stephanie R.*

Hypoglycemia, Dermatitis, Herpes Cold Sores, Sinusitis and Elevated Cholesterol Testimony

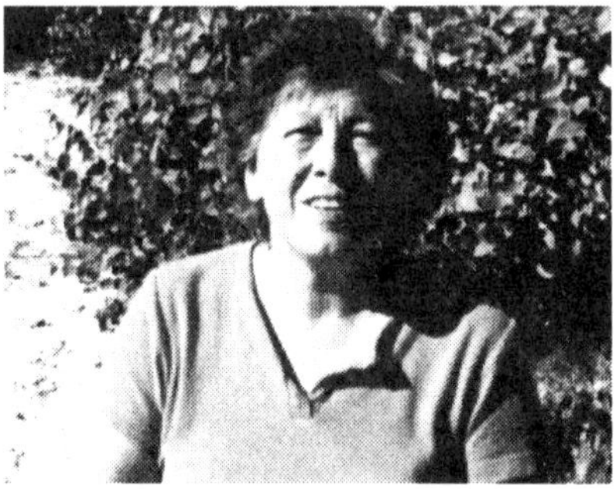

"I am a registered nurse and I would like to tell you about my experience with glyconutritionals. I was having a major health problem; I was having hypoglycemia that was so severe I was quite concerned because I worked in a heart center and in CCU. When your blood sugar drops, then your mental acuity drops, so that was quite serious. I was desperate and looking for something that could help this problem and a friend of mine, Ann, introduced me to these when I needed them. So I looked up the science and all about the nutrients and I said, why not? And so I started taking them and much to my surprise, after three weeks my problem with chronic dermatitis started clearing up. Previously, two dermatologists and the most expensive creams could not do anything for it. And then, as time went on, I had other things happening; but in the meantime I stopped having symptoms and so this was very big for me. I haven't had any more herpes cold sores, my chronic sinusitis is basically gone, my cholesterol dropped 40 points in six months, which I was not even watching but it was found in a routine check-up. I am starting to lose weight, which is a big bonus, and it just goes on and on.

"The eye doctor told me my eyes were in great shape for my age and my dentist also told me that my teeth were really improving, my gums were looking good, and so I have had nothing but positive health benefits and it is so great not to go into diabetes like the endocrinologist told me would happen because diabetes is a terrible, terrible disease and it is rampant in my family. My older sister is on diabetic medication and I have a cousin who died in a diabetic coma. So this was real serious for me and it took a big paradigm shift for me to come away from the health system that I have known for 24 years as a registered nurse and to make this big step and say there is something else out there and I am going to try it."

– *Joy C., R.N.*

“I believe the health of the mitochondria is key to degenerative disease states, perhaps the underlying cause for all chronic degenerative diseases.”

Chapter 8
MEDICAL AND NUTRITIONAL SCIENCE WORKING TOGETHER

The Dietary Supplement Health and Education Act (DSHEA) opened the door for a new class of scientifically proven nutrients called *nutraceuticals.* According to this new law, "**A nutraceutical is any substance that may be considered a food or part of a food and provides medical or health benefits, including the prevention and treatment of disease.**" The government has finally acknowledged "there is a link between the ingestion of certain dietary supplements and the prevention of chronic diseases." This is an actual excerpt from the DSHEA law.

There may be a time and place for allopathic medicine (traditional treatment), but wouldn't it be prudent to become educated to all possible modalities – especially those which are non-invasive and non-toxic – when considering a course of healing? <u>We need to work together, using the best of medical and nutritional science, for all who suffer sub-optimal health.</u> Still, today, most doctors that belong to the church of modern medicine look unfavorably at the doctor who treats without drugs as a heretic because he or she appears to have rejected the sacrament of medicine. Non-drug healers are regarded as belonging to a different religious system and are thought of as quacks, nuts or faddists.[29] Those who turn up their noses at the suggestion of including diet and supplementation in their modality are not only putting their heads in the sand, but they are also putting their patients' very lives at risk. Every year I become increasingly encouraged though, because more and more medical doctors in America, Canada, Australia, United Kingdom and the rest of the world are gaining knowledge in this new science called *glycomics* and the study of these glyconutrients. More and more medical doctors are recommending glyconutritionals with their treatments.

Medical doctors can only do what they are trained to do. Their primary education is in pathology, the study of disease. Why not study health also, and how to have it, and why not be truly what the word *doctor* means – teacher – and teach the patient how to live a more healthy life through diet, nutrition, exercise, etc.? Out of 126 medical colleges, only a handful offers a one-hour course in nutritional science; and it is an elective subject. How can we expect the doctor to prescribe glyconutrients when it is not part of his or her protocol yet, or how can we expect them to even support nutrition when it is not included in the curriculum in medical schools? It is not the doctors' fault, but when you become more proactive in nutrition and your own health or the health of a loved one, the doctors will want to become educated also. For those who do not, I will just say: Condemnation before investigation is the height of arrogance. My advice to all doctors is: <u>Nobody cares how much you know until they know you care enough to diligently check out new information coming from fields other than your own.</u> You might be asking yourself, "Why doesn't my doctor want to know?" It's like going out of the box for your doctor. Their training is largely funded by the drug companies and they are told that foods and supplements are not science, so stick to pharmaceuticals. Basically, it is not profitable for the drug companies. The products are hard to patent and there is not much money to be made in functional foods or supplements. Medical training, couched in pharmaceuticals, has provided us with a range of therapeutics for acute medical emergencies and I appreciate and recognize the tremendous contribution to the health industry. However, the pharmaceutical modality has fostered an unhealthy dependency culture which is built around managing disease usually already in the latter stages when signs and symptoms have become manifested. Medical training should include how to prevent disease and the study of health – not just the study of disease as I said, which is pathology, and a major part of the doctors' curriculum. **The answers for chronic degenerative diseases lie in looking at what makes health, not what causes disease;** this would be a more positive approach. Is the glass half full or half empty? We have many drugs to block, mask, inhibit, suppress and toxify the body, but hardly any cures.

Here is a question for you: If you blow your vehicle's water pump, are you going to replace the vehicle's carburetor in the hope that the water pump will start to work again? Of course not. It is a dumb question; but bear with me a little longer and I will make my point. Obviously, you would replace or rebuild the broken water pump in your vehicle with the same type and configuration that was there and working fine earlier. It would be made of the same materials that the old pump was made of, right? Now, let's look at another vehicle, the one you walk around in, and its pump – the heart. What is it made of? Nostrums, coal tar, petroleum, the stuff many of our drugs are formulated out of? NO, absolutely not! Your heart is made by our Creator, using the best of nutrients, like pure water, proteins, glyconutrients, phytonutrients, phytosterols, vitamins and minerals and other live nutrients. So, if we are going to fix the pump in either vehicle, let's put back the same material that was designed to be there in the first place. You know, I have never seen or heard of any BODY being deficient of any kind of drug. Have you? NEVER! Deficient of nutrients – ABSOLUTELY! So maybe you who are closed-minded might want to re-open your mind and re-think your position and include nutritional support.

Can we conclude that if we have an internal problem with the working parts of the vehicle that we walk around in, that it might be wise to replace the sick and hurting parts with the same kind of material that it is made of? I think it would be logical to restore rather than to treat by masking or blocking symptoms by forcing something foreign and harmful into the vehicle.

I believe there is a place for both schools of science – medical and nutritional. It is called complementary and integrative . . . established medical science and documented nutritional science working together for the benefit of the individuals who are sick and hurting. Dr. Glen Hyland, board certified radiation oncologist and a clinical associate professor of medicine, recounts four particular cancer cases in an interview with the *Grapevine* magazine: "One patient with lung cancer and brain metastases had undergone all the standard radiation and chemotherapy," he explained. "The others were suffering from colon, ovarian and brain cancers. They had all failed standard therapies, including radiation and multiple chemotherapy treatments. Each patient suddenly began showing marked improvement. They experienced weight gain and dramatic reduction in the size of their tumors along with a noticeable increase in their activity levels and a decrease in pain. One of the patients, previously confined to his home, was even able to return to work. Questioning them as to what, if anything, they were doing differently, we found there was a common thread linking them together – they had all begun taking glyconutrients, or dietary supplements we now refer to as 'nutraceuticals.' With four patients showing remarkable results in a six week period, I decided it would be well worth investigating the phenomenon." He went on to say, "While we recognize that these glyconutritional dietary supplements are not manufactured to diagnose, treat or prevent any disease, we are seeing remarkable results when these natural products are introduced into the diets of certain patients." On the last page of the interview, Dr. Hyland said, "The use of these dietary supplements will not replace the treatment and medication patients are on, but rather will work synergistically with them. They will complement each other."[30,31] Hoorah for Dr. Hyland!

Dr. Paul Clayton is a senior lecturer at the Institute of Optimum Nutrition in London, England, and a Royal Society of Medicine Fellow. In an article on July 18, 2002, he said in the *Australian Financial Review,* "One should not fall into the trap of seeking to replace one "magic bullet" with another. Nevertheless, **pharmaco-nutritional programs are poised to do for degenerative diseases what antibiotics did for infectious illnesses, and the potential health care cost savings are enormous**. The social implications of the prospective changes in public morbidity and mortality, which may represent as many as 25 additional healthy middle and old age years will be even more significant."

There is an old saying: "Don't throw the baby out with the bath water." As a nutritionist, I would be doing that very thing if I excluded all modalities of medical science. God forbid you should fall off a roof or get into a serious auto accident, or return home from eating out and suddenly come down with food poisoning. I pray you are rushed to an emergency hospital because in America, when it comes to emergency medical care, we are second to none!

Major Heart Attack and Sinus Problem Testimony

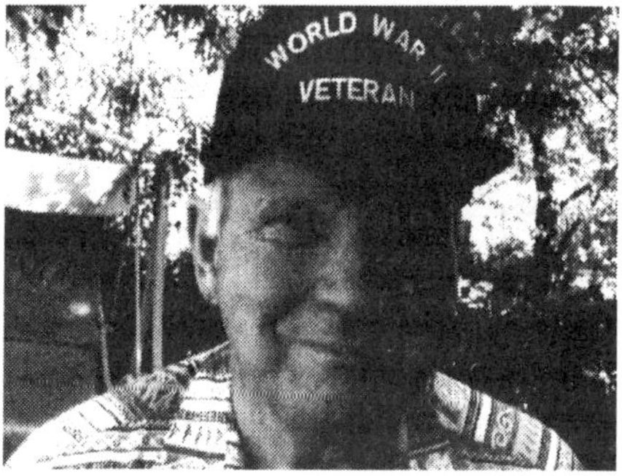

"Twelve years ago I had two major heart attacks. My heart stopped 29 times, 25 of them within 16 hours. The first time I died I was dead for over five minutes and it took them five times to bring me around with electrical shocks. Throughout all of it they used electric shocks on me 34 times to bring me back. I lost the left side of my heart and the right side is now doing all the work. I have been on glyconutritionals now for about six years and I feel great! My energy level is up and I feel good. During the last 35 years I have had sinus problems and the VA tried all kinds of chemicals on me and they couldn't do anything for it. So, since I have used these glyconutritionals and I haven't used any nose spray or anything, and I was hooked on it before. And the Lord Jesus Christ is the one that gave me all the hope and direction and I give him the glory for everything. Dr. Dubouch introduced me to these glyconutritionals and ever since then I have been feeling great and I am still working."

– *Bobby T.*

Lupus Testimony

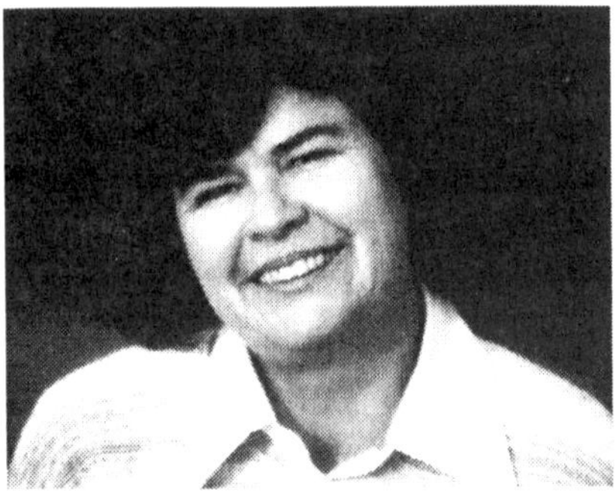

"Back in 1972 I was diagnosed with lupus; they didn't know much about it at that time. They told me there was no cure and they put me on prednisone and Mertruane and pain pills and that was it. They sent me home. I went into remission quite a few times over the years which is typical for lupus, and the last time I came out of remission it was 1995 and it was the worst. I couldn't move, I couldn't walk, I felt like the tin man and when I went to the doctor, they again put me on prednisone and did shocks to my legs and knees and there was nothing to do except to give me their medicine and pain pills. My brother heard how sick I was and sent me some glyconutritionals and told me to take them, and so I did. He would call to check on me regularly and in about three months I was feeling a new sense of well-being. I was able to get up out of the chair and do other things and in six months I was walking and functioning normally. Now I am walking about two miles a day – five miles on a good day. I thank the Lord for that and I thank my brother."

– *Gale B.*

Chapter 9
GLYCONUTRITIONAL LONGITUDINAL TRIALS: A LOOK AT THE RESEARCH

In 1995, the Health and Medical Research Foundation, an independent research organization, began longitudinal trials on the safety and efficacy of the glyconutritionals that I have been discussing in this book. For over 30 years, the foundation has conducted clinical trials for some of the largest nutritional companies in the world. The foundation's Clinical Advisory Board is comprised of internationally known researchers, including professors from major universities, past presidents of the American College of Nutrition and the American College of Sports Medicine. Among other credentials and membership in scientific organizations, the foundation's director, Gilbert R. Kaats, Ph.D., is a lifetime fellow of the American Association of Integrative Medicine as well as a fellow of the American College of Nutrition. He has conducted over 40,000 measurements of body fat and lean during his 30 years of research experience.

Dr. Kaats' research team used pre- and post-study measurements of generally accepted biomarkers of aging and immunity similar to the biomarkers described by Drs. Evans and Rosenberg in their book, *Biomarkers: The 10 Keys to Prolong Vitality* (Simon and Shuster, NYC). The theoretical model the research team used is best illustrated by Drs. Evans and Rosenberg's Disability Zone diagram shown on the next page. The researchers believed that if they could make even small changes in the decline of the average person's health span, it could prolong their years of vitality and well being, thus extending the time at which they would enter the Disability Zone (the point at which one needs to be cared for by someone else).

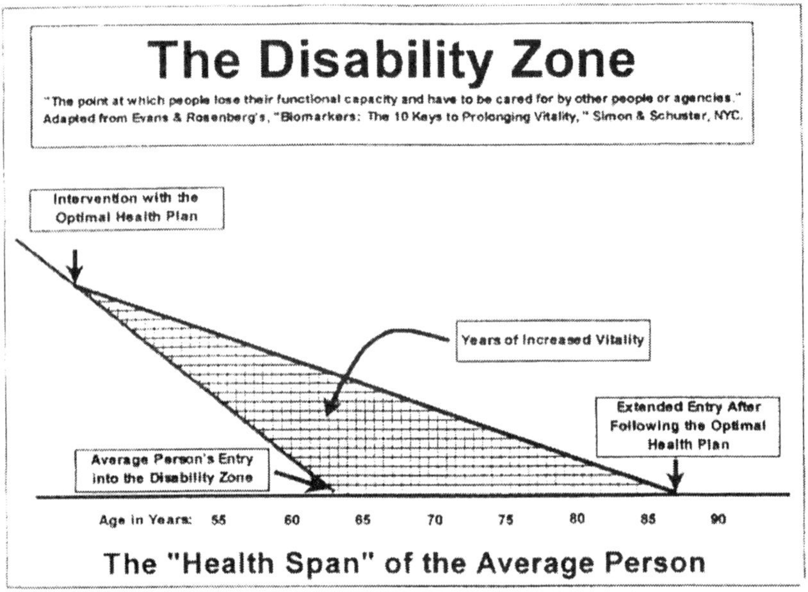

The diagram clearly shows and the data supports that when people add the Optimal Health Plan (glyconutrient complex, phytonutrient complex, phytosterol complex) to their diets and include a physical activity of regular exercise, <u>the years of increased vitality for the average person becomes extended</u>. For information about these three glyconutritionals, go to Appendix A – Product Information.

In 1999, my good friend Frank A. Moore, M.D., and I reviewed the foundation's studies and were impressed not only with the preliminary results, but with the quality of the testing technology the foundation used as well as the credentials of the investigators. We contacted Dr. Kaats and agreed to co-sponsor a leg of the longitudinal trials in our area and serve as co-investigators for the study. We began the study in October of 1999 and completed it in February of 2000. In spite of the fact that conducting clinical trials over the holiday season is the most difficult time of the year to keep people involved, we saw firsthand, as well as through our discussions with Dr. Kaats, the changes that occurred in people using the glyconutritionals and following a behavior modification plan for the 90 days of our study leg.

We had 70 people participate in our study who were tested in the foundation's mobile unit before and after using Dual Energy X-Ray Absorptiometry (DEXA) – the "gold standard" for measurements of bone density, body fat and lean mass.[32,33,34,35] In addition to the DEXA scanner, we included in our leg of the longitudinal trial, a test for arterial elasticity using an FDA-approved CardioVision unit, a test indicator of a person's cardiovascular vessel flexibility. Lack of vessel flexibility has been shown to correlate directly with an increased incidence of heart attacks and strokes. These tests indicate general body health and a direction for correction using glyconutritionals, dietary lifestyle changes and exercise.[36]

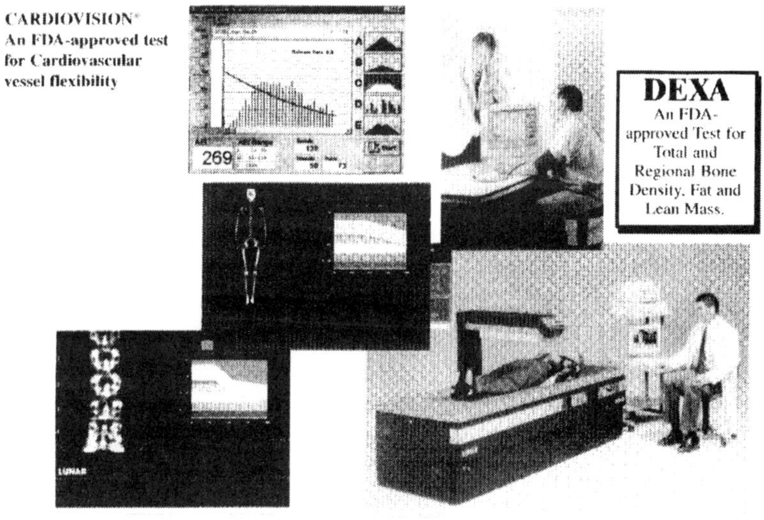

We observed some remarkable individual changes in people who had dramatic increases in bone density, added lean mass, improved their blood chemistries and made quantum leaps in their quality of life. But beyond these personal testimonies, the results of our study leg were consistent with what the researchers were finding in the clinical trials. As a group, study subjects lost fat, preserved lean, increased their bone density, improved their blood chemistries and reported significant improvements on Quality of Life Questionnaires administered at the end of the study.[36,37,38] Thus, the scientific data from an independent team confirmed what Dr.

Moore and I had been seeing for years – glyconutritionals work and work well.[39,40]

As a footnote, the results of the research program's nine-year study have been accepted for publication in the peer-reviewed medical journal, *Advances in Therapy*, which was available at the time my book was being printed, December 2003

.

Osteoporosis Testimony

.

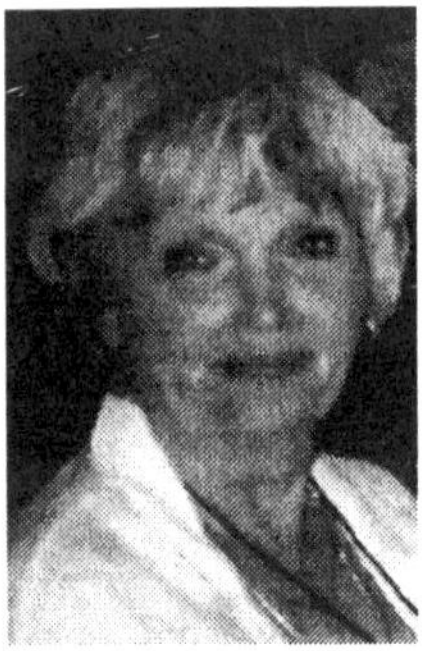

"In 1995 I broke my leg, and when the doctor set it he told me that he had to put two pins in below the knee to hold it together and he said he could have pushed those pins in with his fingers, so that was pretty bad and that scared me a little bit. The doctor had put me on Fosamax which I took for about a month and then I quit because it had some side effects that I didn't like. So I was looking around for some nutrients and I found the glyconutritionals that I began taking at that time.

"I didn't know what would happen, so I didn't know whether it would help my bone mass or not, but I liked the results I was getting anyway. My circulation improved, my coloring improved, my hair texture improved, I was feeling very good; I like to work and it helped me to do a lot of work. I am an artist, so I could stand up all day and paint. And then a number of years later I had another bone scan and I couldn't get any results from the doctor. But about a month ago I had another one done and I went to the hospital and asked absolutely for the paper and I wasn't leaving until I got it. Here I am taking these nutrients and I wanted to find out the results. If I am going to do this, I wanted to know if I am improving or not. So they finally gave it to me and they said I wouldn't understand it. I said, well, that is all right because I have friends (medical doctors). At the bottom of the paper, the testing doctor had written the results for my doctor. It stated that there was significant bone mass improvement since the last bone scan, so I was pretty excited about that.

"I have been on these glyconutritionals for six years; I am 77 years old and of course I prayed all the time and know the Lord has been involved in all of this, and He showed me the way and I am very happy about the whole thing."

– *Dolores R.* (6/18/02) (Maintained bone density and overall good health: 11/27/03)

"Your body knows more about what you need and don't need than all the doctors in the world. We just have to stop assaulting it with what harms and start supplying it with what is missing. Then your body will heal itself."

Chapter 10
THE TRUTH IS OUT

For the last two to three decades, Americans have been sold a bill of goods on low-fat, low-cholesterol diets, resulting in Americans becoming fatter and fatter, blood pressures going higher and higher with degenerative diseases increasing at alarming rates.

Scientific American magazine, January 2003 issue, had an article written by Walter Willet and Meir Stampfer which basically stated, we (meaning established health care and its incorrect food pyramid) have been telling you to eat things that cause you to get fat and causes atherosclerosis and cancer. WE ARE SORRY IT IS THE WRONG STUFF.[41,42] Such recommendations have not provided disease protection but rather contributed to the current epidemics of obesity, heart disease and diabetes as well.

Iain MacRobert, M.D., said in an email letter from his large pediatric practice in Hong Kong:

"In times of physical or emotional stress, and in the absence of a proper dietary intake of the sugars (glyconutrients), the cells do not make proper glycoproteins. Dietary lack therefore results in defective immune response, either too much or too little. Allergic conditions are examples of an over reactive immune system. An under reactive immune system could result in an inability of the natural "killer" cells to recognize diseased or cancerous cells, and dispose of them. The consequence may mean the death of the person. When the cells are given the nutrients they need and they begin to function properly, the resultant health benefits range from profound to amazing. In some cases, the established medical science rules have been overturned. I have spoken to people who had (past tense) multiple sclerosis and who now do not have it. Their neurological lesions have disappeared from the MRI scan. To a natural medical skeptic like myself, the implication of this reversal was simple – medicine is now facing the need for a total paradigm shift in its thinking, as deep a shift as that which occurred when bacteria, and not "bad air," were first shown to be the agents of infectious diseases. The medical profession, myself included, needs to move from a curative view to a wellness view for what we do."

Hepatitis C Testimony

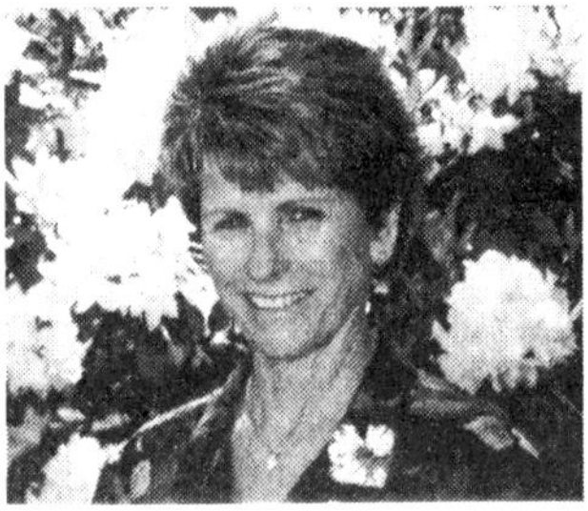

"Thirty years ago I contracted hepatitis C through a blood transfusion, and just in the past three years I started having symptoms. The virus became active and I found myself becoming very fatigued; my body was very weak, my liver enzymes were elevated and eventually my viral load was checked and it was way out of sight. So I underwent interferon treatments and ribvirin, which lasted about seven months; and that type of treatment really wipes you out. I got very ill, but tried to continue to work. The doctor approached me with possibly having another treatment and, boy – that just did not sit well with me and I put that on the shelf for awhile.

"In the meantime, I was approached by my friend Joy, an R.N. at the hospital where I work who knew someone also at work who was involved with glyconutritional supplements. She introduced me to the products and I decided it wouldn't hurt to try it because I definitely did not want to go through treatment again. I started taking several of the products and within a couple of days (I know it wasn't my imagination) I was feeling a lot more energetic and within a couple of weeks I realized that when I went home from work I wasn't falling into bed any more and having to spend my days off in bed trying to re-energize for the rest of the week at work. So I continued to take them and I was really thrilled, needless to say. Within a couple of months I had my viral load tested again and it was non-detectable and I was thrilled and was so thankful to the Lord for bringing me to these people who shared these supplements with me. Since then, which has been almost a year, I have been tested two more times and the viral load remains non-detectable and so you know I am thrilled and it is my desire to share these products with as many people as I can and to get that message out because the Lord is definitely doing the work through these products, I believe."

– Jeri B.

Chapter 11
HOW TO OVERCOME ADD AND ADHD

Many years ago my son was diagnosed with neurological transmitter dysfunction; this is what his doctor, a neurologist, said he had. Today, they call it attention deficit disorder (ADD) or attention deficit hyperactivity disorder (ADHD). Back then when my son was in junior high, the doctor wanted to put him on methylphenidate, commonly known as Ritalin. The protocol is still the same today as it was almost twenty years ago, only now the percentage of children on this drug is outrageous! There are almost six million children in our public schools that are given Ritalin or similar psychotropic agents and anti-depressant drugs like Dexedrine, Prozac and Luvox every day. Our American children consume more of these drugs than all the rest of the children in the world.

In some cases this modality has justification, but six million kids . . . this is an excessive and abusive use of drugs. I can say this because we have had 100 percent success working with parents and doctors to help these children not only to cut back on the drugs, but in most situations, eliminate these drugs completely. Within 90 days of using two or three supplements, mainly a glyconutrient complex and a phytonutrient complex, we have been able to reverse all symptoms of ADD and ADHD. Along with these problems we have seen improvements with oppositional defiant disorder (ODD), conduct disorder (CD) and bipolar problems.

There is a better way – at least one that should be considered before resorting to toxic drugs. **I believe that the greatest crime in the healing arts today is the mindless suppression of symptoms with drugs, especially with our children.**

ADD and ADHD Testimony

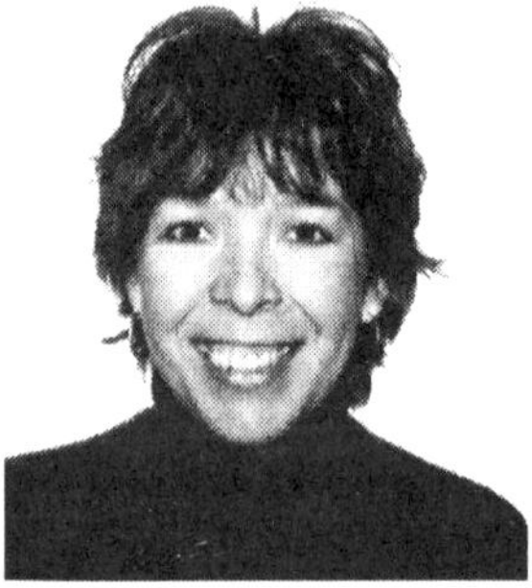

"I have four boys. My two younger boys, Curtis and Wesley, had challenges as soon as they hit the school system. They were diagnosed ADD and ADHD. They go through the obvious things, checking their eyes and their ears, and when they found no problem there, they suggested perhaps my boys needed Ritalin. My story is no different than most; it seems to be a quick-fix that most people reach for. My husband was not going down that road at all with our boys, but I have to tell you, he wasn't the one meeting the teacher in the hallway every day hearing them tell about the bad day my child was having at school. It was taking its toll on me personally, and especially with Curtis. He is nine years old this year and this has been going on for several years. Curtis would come home from school saying things like, 'I don't know why I was born,' 'I'm stupid,' 'I have no purpose.' Hearing this just broke my heart.

"I didn't know how to help him other than using the drugs. The teacher said there were kids that are getting help that are on this Ritalin; so I was ready. I wanted them to give me Prozac and Ritalin for my son – anything that could help him. My husband, of course, didn't want to do that. So we started searching further for a solution – a natural, non-drug solution. We tried the health food store thing and spent a lot of money there, but had little or no results. Then we found these glyconutrients and phytonutrients and I purchased a small amount. We started out slow because I wanted to see a little improvement before I spent any more money. I've got to be honest with you, I was very surprised. I saw results the next day. The teacher met me in the hall and said, "What have you done with

Curtis?" Besides giving our boys these glyconutrients, we had to take a closer look at what they were eating, i.e., sugar, junk foods, etc. Curtis used to suck and chew on his shirtsleeves and collars. They would be soaking wet and there were bite marks on all of his clothes. All of this stopped once he started taking the glyconutritional products. He has no bad behaviors, none of the symptoms, no ticks, nothing. His attitude is wonderful and he even feels good about himself now.

"My younger son, Wesley, has more of the hyperactivity that is involved with ADHD. I've had a little more of a challenge with him, but over the course of a year, we are miles ahead of where we were last year. The boys are in a new school and the teachers have never seen them without these products. They have no idea of how they were before, but the difference is like night and day. I am now working with other families, helping them, and we are seeing remarkable changes. If you have a child suffering with a similar problem, know that they are really very smart, but they feel so stupid. It's criminal what is happening to these kids on drugs. We have to help them and share the knowledge of good nutrition and these glyconutritionals. The children do not have a learning disability. The products supply missing nutrients the body needs to correct the problem. This is not magical, but it's just that we don't eat properly and most of the food we eat is unacceptable for good health. We will never be without these products. My husband and I highly recommend them."

– Katherine O.

Ritalin is a Class II drug, the same as cocaine and morphine. Be aware that if your child takes this drug past the age of 12, according to the 1999 Military Recruitment Manual your child may not join any military organization (Army, Navy, Air Force or Marines). Not ever! Your child will be classified as a Class II drug user.

The state and federal government cannot hire your child if the job involves state secrets or national security because your child is a Class II drug user. Some insurance companies will turn down someone for being a Class II drug user; others will raise their rates and write in a pre-existing condition clause. Ritalin has similar side effects as those of cocaine because the two are almost identical chemical compounds. Studies strongly suggest that children with ADHD are at significantly higher risk for antisocial- and substance-related disorders in adulthood.

I have many documented stories of the tragic consequences of taking these horrific drugs to support my case for a natural, safe approach. Here are just a few. On May 25, 1997, 18-year-old Jeremy Strohmeyer raped and murdered a 7-year-old girl in Las Vegas, Nevada. Strohmeyer had been diagnosed with ADD and prescribed Dexedrine, a Ritalin-like drug, immediately prior to the killing.

On October 1, 1997 in Pearl, Mississippi, 16-year-old Luke Woodham stabbed his mother to death and then went to his high school where he shot nine people, killing two teenage girls and wounding seven others. Published reports say he was on Prozac.

Exactly two months later, on December 1, 1997, Michael Carneal, a 14-year-old, opened fire on students at a high school prayer meeting in West Paducah, Kentucky. You might remember hearing about the incident on the radio or TV. Three teenagers were killed, five others were wounded, one of whom was paralyzed. Michael was reportedly on Ritalin.

This story was on all the major news media and happened on May 21, 1998, when 15-year-old Kip Kinkel, of Springfield, Oregon, murdered his parents and proceeded to his high school where he went on a rampage, killing 2 students and wounding 22 others. Kip had been prescribed both Ritalin and Prozac.

Here is just one more terrible story that happened in Colorado in 1999. It also was highly televised. Eighteen-year-old Eric Harris killed twelve students and a teacher at Columbine High School before killing himself. Harris was on one of the anti-depressants called Luvox. Ninety percent of the children involved in the recent serial killings were taking properly prescribed mind-altering drugs. Was this fact reported by the major media at the time? Do you remember any comments regarding the above five stories and the drugs these kids were on? If not, why not?

If your school board's regulations recommend putting your child on one of these drugs, do not be intimidated into thinking that they have the only solution. Get help, but do not jump onto the drugging bandwagon that many schools advocate. If they tell you, "The law says if your child is disruptive in class you have to put the child on Ritalin," ask them to show you the law in writing. The law will usually say that if your child is physically endangering other children, then you must seek medical help or special classes, and even then, that does not always mean drugs. If they tell you to sign a release for your child's medical records because it is the law, again ask to see the law in writing. You are the parent; you raise your children. They are the school board, and they deal in education. Let's keep it that way.

Whenever you go before a review board or conference regarding your child, record the meeting on a tape recorder – not hidden, but in plain sight. Explain that you cannot take notes and listen at the same time because you want to remember every word they say. If they say the meeting is private and confidential and cannot be recorded, ask them to put that in writing. <u>You are never in a closed-door session regarding your children.</u>

Benjamin Rush, M.D., a signer of the Declaration of Independence and personal physician to George Washington, said: "Unless we put medical freedom into the Constitution, the time will come when medicine (and the drug cartel) will organize into an undercover dictatorship to restrict the art of healing to one class of men and deny equal privilege to others: the Constitution of the Republic should make a special privilege for medical freedoms as well as religious freedom." Non-toxic, safe natural modalities that have scientific validation should be allowed in the same arena as allopathic medicine (traditional treatment), the same as it is in Europe.

I elaborated on ADD and ADHD specifically because of the problem my son had. This is where my heart is – with the innocent and helpless children.

Chapter 12
DIFFERING MODELS OF HEALTH

My friend Marcia Smith, N.D., Ph.D., wrote a paper explaining the military disease model and the terrain model very succinctly, so I thought it would be a valuable addition to this publication. Dr. Smith's beautiful explanation gives credence to what I call the metabolic glyconutritional discovery. Dr. Marcia Smith holds three degrees: a master's degree and Ph.D. in holistic nutrition and a degree as a Doctor of Naturopathy. She currently lectures throughout the United States, Canada and the United Kingdom.

[Reprinted by permission.]

The Military, Disease Model

The prevailing model for health in the West is the military, disease model – a model of "divide and conquer." Western medicine divides the body into systems, parts (organs) and functions, and it treats these separate aspects as if they were not part of a whole. Medicine frequently names diseases by translating the name of the body part and the dysfunction of that part into Latin or Greek (or both). For instance, the word "arth" means joint, and "itis" means inflammation. So arthritis literally means, "inflamed joint." When you tell the doctor that your joint hurts, he/she essentially translates what you have told him/her into another language and diagnoses "arthritis." A diagnosis allows a doctor to decide which medication would be necessary to control, manipulate, kill, or suppress a system or function. This model looks at the various parts of the body as being "enemies." Doctors speak of "controlling" a disease. They speak of the "war on cancer" or the "war on heart disease." Their medications are referred as their "armamentarium" (their chest of weapons). They speak of looking for the "magic bullet." Their language is evidence of their mindset. The goal of the military model is often the "quick fix." The goal is to "fight" now; worry about the "debris" later. People readily "feel" the effects of the Western approach when their pain is turned off or symptoms are suppressed. There is often the appearance of health, but that appearance is often transitory. The substance of health is frequently missing.

This model has worked well with crisis care. Western medicine has the best system in the world for dealing with life-threatening infections, sophisticated surgeries, and the like. However, it is a fact that chronic, degenerative diseases (statistically those from which most of us will die) have become the most common problems that medicine currently faces, and those diseases are on the rise. Heart disease is up 400 percent since 1900; diabetes is up 700 percent since 1959; and cancer is projected to surpass heart disease as the #1 killer in less then 20 years. I believe that there is no evidence that the military model will save us from chronic, degenerative disease.

Along with being powerless to deal with chronic, degenerative diseases, the military approach is also powerless to deal with the emergence of autoimmune diseases in the twentieth century. Autoimmune diseases have brought great frustration to Western medicine because no external "bad guy" has been identified. Instead, the body itself has become the "bad guy" because it is attacking itself. In the presence of an autoimmune condition, the Western medical approach suppresses the body's own immune system with anti-inflammatory drugs. This often produces symptomatic relief, but it does not address the underlying reason why the body is harming itself. Without dealing with the cause, there is little likelihood of finding real healing. As you can see, the military model has failed to solve the problems of most modern diseases. So, where did the military model come from?

The Terrain Model

The history of medicine shows that the military model emerged after Pasteur's discovery of disease organisms as the cause of disease. In Pasteur's day, a different model had many advocates – the model of improving the "terrain" of the body. Terrain literally means "soil." It was observed that numerous individuals had survived various plagues. There was an understanding that their survival was no accident, and it was believed that their survival related to their overall healthy constitution. At that time the focus of medicine was to find elements necessary to build a healthy constitution and thereby build health. The perception that the quality of the constitution was related to health was recently reiterated by a well-known twentieth-century immunologist, Dr. Rangit Chandra.

He found an interesting correlation between the occurrence of plagues and famines in Medieval Europe. By studying death records and graveyards, he found that plague repeatedly and predictably followed famine. Those that famine touched got nutritionally weaker (as the "terrain" got weaker) from famine-induced malnutrition. Their likelihood of dying from plague grew stronger. Those not affected by the famine survived.

Unfortunately, since the time of Pasteur, the discovery of disease organisms has become so fascinating that interest in looking at the "terrain" has virtually ceased. This is especially unfortunate since it has been reported that even Pasteur, on his deathbed, recanted his belief that the disease organism was primary, and said, "The terrain is everything."

How does this discussion relate to nutraceuticals and specifically glyconutrients, phytonutrients and phytosterols?

These supplements are "rooted" (pun intended) in the "terrain" model. It is important that you fully understand this model in order to comprehend the answers you seek regarding these products. It is helpful to first understand the meaning of "terrain."

The model of the "terrain" or "soil" is an agricultural model instead of a military model. The best way to describe it is to give an overview of how agriculture has worked successfully for thousands of years.

Any farmer, pre-1945, knew that healthy plants grew from healthy soil. The practice of rotating crops, leaving fields fallow, using compost and organic fertilizers served to keep the soil healthy. Additionally, damage from "pests" and plant disease were minimized by having healthy plants which could resist these threats. After 1945, especially in the U.S., there was a shift toward "agribusiness" with the appearance of large farms utilizing chemical fertilizers designed to produce "bumper crops." "Old-fashioned" methods were abandoned, and the large-scale application of chemical pesticides and herbicides was implemented. The focus became production of food in great quantity, to the neglect of quality in terms of nutritional value.

The traditional methods of farming are the basis of current methods of organic farming. Healthy plants require minimal use of chemicals to handle the "pests." If needed, natural methods are the chosen remedy (such as introducing ladybugs and praying mantis). Great attention is paid to the health of the soil – its proper pH and its mineral balance. For instance, many organic gardeners utilize pulverized glacial rock in order to re-mineralize the soil. Rebuilding the soil is a long, careful, and expensive process. Many feel that it is worth the trouble. There is certainly no need for genetic engineering on an organic farm.

Applying the Agricultural Model to the Body

Applying the agricultural model to the body is really quite simple. As the "terrain" of our bodies is altered through deficiencies in basic nutrients (essential vitamins, minerals, amino acids, fatty acids, carbohydrates – especially the eight monosaccharides needed for glycoconjugate synthesis), our organs and systems become weaker (like weak plants). The body is also weakened by having to handle an unprecedented number of toxins from the water, the air, and the food. As a result of being weakened, various organisms such as viruses, bacteria, yeasts, or parasites have taken over our bodies, just as the "pests" have taken over the weak plants grown on devitalized soil. In this farming analogy, Western medicines become the "pesticides," focused on killing the bad organisms. When those medicines don't work to solve the problem, the genetic engineers come in to manipulate the genes in our bodies – just as the genetic engineers are trying to do in agriculture in order to manipulate the genes in our plants. The metaphor is both accurate and "chilling."

The Search for Alternatives

Many individuals are sensing that the Western medical model is not working. They are confused as to where to turn. In this search many are seeking alternative care. In their search for answers they have found intelligent and caring doctors who are turning to "natural medicine." Others are walking the aisles of health food stores, filling their baskets with the items from advertisements and articles in health magazines. I find that in both situations they are coming away with bags full of dietary supplements, which, in some cases, produce only limited results. Many of those individuals have found their way to nutritionists familiar with these glyconutritionals, and have subsequently found greater success on a few of these products, than they did with bags of other supplements. What is the difference? How can that be? My perception is that most "natural doctors" are still practicing the "divide and conquer" model of healing – they are just using natural substances for "bullets" instead of using drugs. They are, for instance, using anti-viral nutrients or herbs, or specific substances that work on certain immune cells. They are still dividing the person up into parts, organs, and cells, and they are treating those parts separately (usually at great cost to the patient). I don't see most of them looking at the "terrain." Health magazines tout the latest remedies for this or that problem. From reading these articles, you would think that you should be taking them ALL. Although these approaches are often better (and certainly less toxic) than using drugs, they are still not generally working to balance the "terrain" in an organized and optimal way. I find that if you are not working to balance the "terrain" first, you will not have maximum success.

I, myself, used to practice in this fashion (using lots of nutrients and herbs focused on different systems and organs). The results I had were nothing compared to what I have had using the spectrum of these glyconutritional products as the foundation first.

The Optimal Health Plan (glyconutrient, phytonutrient and phytosterol) provides key nutrients for the body – food that has been removed by the modern lifestyle. The science behind this glyconutrient complex is revolutionary, and I am thrilled to be involved in a breakthrough in health. Although the carbohydrates in this glyconutrient have not been officially and legally defined as "essential," I believe they should be. It is my belief that this glyconutrient is a crucial blend of nutrients for repairing the body's "terrain." Its potential for normalizing cell-to-cell communication is an essential element in "terrain" building. Cell-to-cell communication plays a major part of the body's recognition of itself, thus minimizing the body's self-destruction.

These products are proprietary (because of the patent-pending status of this glyconutrient complex), and they can't be duplicated by another company. No substitute will do. No substitute exists! All of these supplements are providing a balance of nutrients necessary for building health through rebuilding the "terrain" of the body. Re-balancing the soil of an organic farm does not require the use of a single nutrient, and no one nutrient is more important than another. Careful attention is required to provide a blend of nutrients that work synergistically. It takes TIME for the natural balance to return. It requires the practice of patience and careful attention to the progress being made.

Rebuilding the body "terrain" also requires that you look at the quality of the food you eat, the liquids that you drink. You also need to look at the metabolic effect of certain foods, choosing primarily those that will not raise your blood sugar quickly (low-glycemic foods). You need to minimize your exposure to toxins (synthetic chemicals) in your food and airborne toxins in your home. You need enough rest – just as sometimes fields need to lie fallow for a period of time. Your emotions affect your "terrain," and keeping them in a healthy balance can also have a major effect on your overall health.

It takes TIME to rebuild your health, just as it takes time to rebuild the soil in an organic garden. People may not immediately feel the changes that are taking place. They are subtle and incremental. The body is programmed towards health when the "terrain" is healthy just as plants are programmed to grow into vital and healthy foods in the proper soil. Listening to your body is important.

This does not mean that you would never take a medication again. Medications definitely have their place in crisis care. Also, if you have been prescribed medications, you need to stay on them while gradually rebuilding the "terrain." As your body moves in the direction of health, you should only taper off medications under the guidance of a pharmacist trained to understand these glyconutritionals or your medical doctor who is knowledgeable in this new science called nutraceuticals.

Marcia Smith, N.D., Ph.D.

Author's Comment: How do you treat a sick fish? You treat the terrain – the water the fish is swimming in!

Chapter 13
REDUCE YOUR FEAR OF BIOTERRORISM

One of the major health concerns that has recently developed is the threat of attack by terrorists using chemical and biological weapons. In November, 2001, at the U.S. House Government Reform Committee hearing, Chairman, Congressman Dan Burton (R-IN), held a full committee hearing entitled "Comprehensive Medical Care for Bioterrorism Exposure." The panel consisted of a Major General from the Army Medical Research Institute for Infectious Diseases, a representative from the Department of Defense and M.D.s and Ph.D.s from various other agencies. The hearing was covered on C-Span television. H. Reg McDaniel, M.D., one of the presenters, whose topic was "Evidence Supporting the Potential for Glyconutrients and Micronutrient Dietary Supplementation to Support Natural Defense and Healing Mechanisms to Ameliorate Bacterial, Viral and Fungal Infections." As part of his testimony he was asked, ". . . to provide an outline of nutritional issues relating to improving immune response and possible nutritional solutions to complement treatments for most biologic agents." In the executive summary of this hearing it said: **". . . [glyconutrients] are predicted to be effective against war-grade modified organisms, bacterial and viral."**[43] More research was discussed to prove this preventative and therapeutic approach that could be designed to thwart bioterrorism infectious agents which are designed to destabilize the society of America and its allies.

The purpose of the hearing was to review the medical options available to deal with bioterrorism exposure. They discussed how current knowledge has changed as a result of the anthrax exposure. Discussions included nutrition and complementary treatments and what vaccines and antibiotics could be used against biological agents such as anthrax and smallpox. Questions were raised about which antibiotics offered the fewest side effects and whether large-scale use of antibiotics would promote antibiotic-resistant bacteria. No governmental response to Dr. McDaniel's proposal has transpired.

Health officials estimate that there are up to 20,000 cases of antibiotic-resistant infections annually. Many health officials view them as a harbinger of worse to come. Bacteria develop resistance to antibiotics because they evolve so rapidly, two or three times an hour. If a few bacteria develop genes that can protect them from antibiotics, those few resistant microbes can become millions overnight.

You have heard it said, "forewarned is forearmed"; but the major media have decided that scaring people with predictions of chemical and biological warfare makes good news. Omitting important *balancing* facts that would water down and diminish the news stories apparently is not cost effective for the media (the more viewers, listeners and readers, the more money is made). I am grateful for the media in general for keeping us informed, but this is one area where a more balanced view needs to be presented. These news stories should not be all that doom and gloom, and, yes, we should be concerned; but not become panicky. Panic is brought on by fear. Here is what Wordsworth wrote about fear: "What are fears but voices awry? Whispering harm where harm is not. And deluding the unwary."

In the mid-1990s there was a series of nerve gas attacks on crowded Japanese subway stations. Given there were perfect conditions for the attacks, less than 10 percent of the people were harmed and most of them were okay within a few hours. Only one percent of the injured died. This made big news, even here in America. I don't mean to minimize or make light of the incidents; the perpetrators (murderers) should be appropriately dealt with. These weapons are about terror; but if you keep your immune system in good condition, remain calm and listen to the proper authorities, you will be giving yourself a fighting chance. I believe this to be far less scary than the media portrays. Serious, yes – boot-shaking scary, no. There are things *you can do* to protect yourself against chemical and biological terrorism.

Chemical Weapons

Chemical weapons are categorized as nerve, blood and blister incapacitating agents. Contrary to the hype of reporters, they are not weapons of mass destruction. They are "area denial" and terror weapons. When you leave the area that is infected, you almost always leave the risk. These are not gasses; they are vapors and/or airborne particles. The agent must be delivered in sufficient quantity to injure or kill, and that defines when and how it is used. Since they are vapors and airborne particles, these nerve agents are heavier than air, so they will seek low places like ditches, basements and underground garages. The toxins, for the most part, will not be effective when it is cold (freezing) and it does not last long when the temperature is high (hot) and the wind spreads it too thinly and too fast. It almost has to be dumped on you, or you have to directly inhale it for it to cause any serious damage. The concentration of chemicals has to be quite high to kill you unless, of course, your immune system is already compromised and weak. If exposed, your best protection is to stay calm and get out of the area and into fresh air.

Nerve Agents

Some of the symptoms from exposure to chemical nerve agents are sudden headache, dimness of vision (if the person you are looking at has pinpointed pupils), difficulty breathing, runny nose, excessive saliva or drooling, tightness in the chest, stomach cramps, a twitching of the exposed skin where a liquid has made contact. If you are in a public place and you start experiencing these symptoms, ask yourself: Did anything out of the ordinary just happen, like a loud pop, or did someone spray something on the crowd? Are other people getting sick? Is there an odor of newly mowed hay, green corn, something fruity or camphor where it shouldn't be? If the answer is yes, then *calmly* (if you panic, you breathe faster and inhale more air and consequently more poison) leave the area and head upwind or outside. The quickest antidote is fresh air. If you have a blob or splash of liquid on you that looks like molasses or Karo syrup, scrape or blot it off and get it away from you with anything disposable.

Blood Agents

Blood agents are cyanide or ricin which affect your blood's ability to carry and provide oxygen to your tissue. The scenario for attack would be the same as nerve agents. Look for a pop or someone splashing or spraying something and people around you getting woozy and falling down. The telltale smells are bitter almonds or garlic where it would not be expected. The symptoms are blue lips, blue under the fingernails, rapid breathing. Fresh air as soon as possible is your best antidote.

Blister Agents

Blister agents (distilled mustard) are so nasty that nobody even wants to handle them, much less use them. Because it is almost impossible to handle safely and may have delayed effects of up to 12 hours, the attack scenario is also limited to the things you would see from other chemicals. If you *do* get large, painful blisters for no apparent reason, do not pop them. If you must, be very careful not to let the liquid under the blister get on any other area of your body, as the toxic substance will continue to spread. It is just as likely to harm the user as the target. Soap, water, sunshine and fresh air are this toxic substance's enemy.

The bottom line on chemical weapons is that they are intended to make you panic, to terrorize you, to herd you like sheep to the wolves. You are *more* likely to be hurt by a drunk driver on any given day than be hurt by one of these attacks.

Biological Weapons

Biological weapons are vectored (any organism that is the carrier of disease-producing viruses) in bugs and rodents, from one person to another, and with contaminated material. Keep the garbage in your environment to a minimum externally and internally. Do not leave standing, stagnant water (such as in ditches or unused kiddie pools) around to provide breeding room for mosquitoes. Basic personal hygiene and sanitation will go a long way toward preventing an environment that is conducive to these vectors. A healthy immune system is your very best defense and the nutraceuticals (glyconutrient complex, phytonutrient complex and phytosterol complex) are prime nutrients needed by the body to build a healthy immune system. If, after all I have said on this matter, you still want a gas mask, go get one; but I am not getting one. Terrorist weapons are made to cause panic, terror and to demoralize us. If we do not run around like scared-to-death sheep and do not give in to media-hyped isolated incidents, the terrorist will not get much mileage out of his or her crime and will become discouraged and quit. I want to thank retired military expert Red Thomas for his input on this nasty bioterrorism business.

On June 20, 2002, the Center for Disease Control (CDC) held a meeting with the Advisory Committee for Immunization Practices (ACIP). The subject, decisions and testimonies were on the recommendations for smallpox vaccination currently being considered by the CDC and Department of Health and Human Services (DHHS). For some reason, major news media neglected to report on this important meeting. What has come to light because of this and other meetings on a similar subject are the four generally accepted facts about smallpox that *are all wrong!* Here are the four myths:

Myth #1: Smallpox is highly contagious.

Joel Kuritsky, M.D., Director of the National Immunization Program and Early Smallpox Response and Planning at the CDC, said: "Smallpox has a slow transmission and is **not highly contagious**." This is an obvious contradiction to what we have been told about smallpox.

The symptoms after contracting the disease do not occur immediately. It has an incubation period of 3 to 17 days; the first of several symptoms will be the development of a high fever (101°F. or higher). This would be accompanied by nausea, headache, severe abdominal cramping and vomiting, and also low back pain and a rash.

An infected person is not contagious, even with a fever. Not until a rash appears (in two to four days) is a person contagious. The characteristics of the rash are not difficult to diagnose, says Walter A. Orenstein, M.D., Director of the National Immunization Program (NIP) at the CDC. The smallpox rash is a round, firm pustule. The lesions can develop over the entire body but appear to manifest more often on the soles of the feet, on the face and on the palms.

<u>Myth #2</u>: Smallpox can be spread by casual contact with an infected individual.

Smallpox will not spread rapidly, even after the development of a rash. When it does spread, it is usually because the infected person sneezed or coughed directly on another individual. Dr. Orenstein said, "Smallpox will not spread like wildfire; the spread of smallpox to casual contacts is the exception to the rule." The transmission of smallpox occurs only after close, constant exposure, within a few feet of each other for about a week of steady contact.

Dr. Tom Mack, from the University of Southern California, said, "In Pakistan 27 percent of cases demonstrated no transmission to close associates. Nearly 37 percent had a transmission of only one generation." The second person contracting smallpox did not infect anyone else. This is a direct contradiction to the predicted spreading to the millions.

Dr. Kuritsky said at the CDC's public forum on smallpox on June 8, 2002, in St. Louis, Missouri: "Given the slow transmission rate and that people need to be in close contact for nearly a week to spread the infection, the scenario in which a terrorist could infect himself with smallpox and contaminate an entire city by walking through the streets touching people is purely fiction."

<u>Myth #3</u>: There is no known treatment for smallpox.

A more correct statement would be that there are no pharmaceutical drugs for the treatment of smallpox. There are about 300 antiviral drugs and they are testing one that is used for HIV patients. It is very potent and the potential side effects could be extensive. A more natural, safe and effective approach would be to use the metabolic glyconutritional discovery, utilizing all three nutraceuticals (glyconutrient complex, phytonutrient complex, phytosterol complex). H. Reg McDaniel, M.D., said, "Research on this safe, economical, potentially effective approach is warranted."

Myth #4: The smallpox vaccine will prevent a person from getting infected.

There is no clinical proof that vaccines are effective. Vaccines have never been scientifically proven to prevent anyone from getting smallpox. Dr. Harold Margolis, Senior Advisor to the Director for Smallpox Planning and Response, said in Atlanta: "The vaccine decreased the death rate among those vaccinated by modifying the disease, not by preventing infection." Neutralizing antibodies are reported to reflect levels of protection, although this has not been validated in the field.

I think we should be very careful in accepting inoculations of dangerous ineffective experimental vaccines. A national massive smallpox vaccination campaign could set the stage for a health disaster. According to the world health records in England, Germany, Italy, the Philippines, British India, etc., devastating epidemics followed mass vaccination. The worst smallpox disaster occurred in the Philippines after a 10-year compulsory vaccination program. Ten million people were vaccinated, resulting in 170,000 cases of infection and more than 75,000 deaths from smallpox in a country having only scattered cases in rural villages prior to the onslaught of vaccines.

Think about this also: If the terrorists have biological smallpox, what is the chance that they have other weapons of biological destruction . . . those for which we do not have a vaccine? The government *does* have many different kinds of vaccines, but are we going to be subjected and injected with all of them? Did you know that the toxic mercury in most vaccines is dozens of times in excess of the EPA safety levels? Did you know that all 696,000 Gulf War personnel were inoculated with 3 completely untested vaccines, resulting in 80,000 of them contracting a disease known as Gulf War Syndrome? Vaccines are not thoroughly tested before they are put on the market and American children are the most vaccinated group, not only in the world, but in all of history. Does the fact that vaccines are a multi-billion dollar business in the United States have any bearing on what's happening here?

In an editorial, the National Vaccine Information Center (NVIC) co-founder and president, Barbara Loe Fisher, criticizes a federal plan urging state health officials to use the state "militia" to arrest, imprison and force vaccination and medication on Americans and then to be exempt from liability for any injury or death that results. The proposed legislation would also give health officials control of all roads and the power to seize homes, cars, telephones, firearms, supplements and even food. It has already been introduced in Massachusetts. Get educated and spread the word that our freedoms are under attack NOW! The NVIC (http://www.nvic.org) serves as a consumer watchdog on vaccine development and policymaking. NVIC advocates the institution of safety and informed consent protections in the mass vaccination system. They also advocate basic science research into genetic and other biological factors which place some individuals at high risk for vaccine injury and death.

To stay healthy and protected, follow some basic common sense responses to an attack, listen to the proper authority and stay calm; don't listen to hysterical people and don't cower down to news stories of pending doom. Y2K predictions of disasters never happened, but if you got somewhat prepared, you are all the better for it. Yes, forewarned is forearmed, whether it is for smallpox, SARS or any potential problem. Realize that you are not helpless. There are positive things you can do to protect yourself and your loved ones.

You have two major defensive postures you can take. First, is to stay away from infected people and stay clear of infected areas. That is not always possible, but it would be prudent. The second is to stay healthy by keeping your immune system healthy. As I said in the beginning of the book: <u>If you catch the flu easily or often, if you are run down, if you are under constant stress, you worry a lot, you are in a state of depression, you don't sleep well, you feel weak or high strung (explode easily), then your immune system could be compromised. This is especially true if you have a constantly low level of energy.</u> These are red flags, and if you have two or more of these symptoms, it might be wise to contact a nutritionally oriented medical doctor, naturopath, chiropractor, or nutritionist who is familiar with and utilizes nutraceuticals, and particularly glyconutritionals.

The scientist and microbiologist, Dr. Kanatjan Alibekov, developed some of the most heinous biological weapons known to mankind, including the world's most deadly strain of anthrax. The doctor was seeking a remedy for his years of creating weapons of mass destruction. So, in 1999, the CIA helped Dr. Alibek (the name I believe he now uses) to defect from the Soviet Union to the United States. Dr. Alibek is now helping the U.S. find ways to defend against bioweapons. He says, "In the event of an attack, hormones inhaled or injected could quickly fortify the immune system against many different pathogens."

The doctor is on the right track; your best defense is supporting and building up the immune system. Our phytosterol complex (sometimes referred to as phytogenins or phytohormones) is a precursor to the mother hormone dehydroepiandrosterone (DHEA). This would be a perfect nutrient to accompany the glyconutrient complex and phytonutrient complex. I would not be surprised if Dr. Alibek agreed. There is no substitute for the plant phytosterol, which is much safer, compared to taking a synthetic DHEA hormone. There is a correlation between low DHEA levels in the body and degenerative diseases. Julian Whitaker, M.D., states in his *Health and Healing Newsletter*: "DHEA is the closest we can get to the fountain of youth." I think it definitely helps. Scientific research reveals that adequate DHEA in the body can slow the aging process, preventing, and even reversing, disease conditions. Taking these three nutraceuticals together is the metabolic glyconutritional discovery that will do more to build and balance your immune system beyond anything else on the market, according to my research.

Dr. Alibek is an expert scientist on anthrax and other bioterrorism agents. He acknowledges that treating these pathogens with antibiotics is not the best answer. In the event terrorists bioengineer an anthrax organism to resist antibiotics or in case antibiotic supplies are exhausted during an epidemic, there must be some other recourse. He believes the best defense is a healthy immune system.

In my opinion, the best antiviral against anthrax, West Nile virus, SARS, smallpox or any life-threatening microorganism is taking the basic three glyconutritionals I have been writing about here.

I have elaborated on each of these nutraceuticals on the Product Information pages in Appendix A.

This can be a terrifying world we live in today; we are constantly hearing about wars, the dangers of nuclear weapons, chemical and biological terrorism, about earthquakes, floods, hurricanes, tornadoes, global warming and ozone depletion. Diseases are on the rise and crime is prevalent throughout the country. If you want to worry and make yourself sick, there are plenty of reasons – and I am sure you can think of more as well. But, in the midst of it all, God promises to be a refuge and a fortress to those who will trust and dwell in Him. "A thousand shall fall at thy side, and ten thousand at thy right hand; but it shall not come nigh thee. There shall no evil befall thee, neither shall any plague come nigh thy dwelling." (Psalm 91:7,10) He made that promise thousands of years ago to those who believe, when man had not even invented weapons to destroy thousands of people all at once. Today, these calamities are possible and a real threat; but God wants to be your protector and the first name you call on when trouble beseeches you. He is our shelter and refuge. (Refuge means we are inaccessible to the enemy.) No matter how terrifying things around you seem to be, call on Him and trust God. Pray for wisdom and discernment, and by all means, have faith. Seek His guidance; then peace, health and long life will be yours.

Chapter 14
GLYCOBIOLOGY HITS THE BIG TIME

Just as I was finishing work on this book, I received this breaking news cover story, "Ten Technologies That Will Change the World," published in MIT's magazine *Technology Review*, and felt I should add the highlights regarding one of the ten technologies – glycobiology. MIT describes glycobiology as the burgeoning science of glycomics research on sugars and their impact on human health.

In the February 2003 edition of *Technology Review*, the Massachusetts Institute of Technology (MIT) profiled the science of glycomics as a new technology that "...could have an impact on health problems ranging from rheumatoid arthritis to the spread of cancer cells." Glycomics is the study of sugars and includes glycobiology – the study of the effects of sugars on living organisms that is the basis of glyconutritional research and products.

The article detailed at least six scientific experts who are hard at work, trying to synthesize the thousands of sugars made by the human body. These researchers are funded mostly by pharmaceutical companies that hope to turn these sugars into drugs that will boost the immune system and heal disease.

"The reason for the excitement around glycomics is that sugars have a vital function in the body," the article explained. "By manipulating...sugars themselves, researchers hope to shut down disease processes, create new drugs and improve existing ones."

Not an Easy Task

The article also explains that because there's no simple "code" that determines sugar structure, the researchers admit they have an enormous task ahead. They estimate that as many as forty thousand genes make up each person, and each gene can code for several proteins. In fact, sugars modify many of these proteins. Then various cell types attach the same sugars in different ways, forming a variety of branching structures, each with a unique function. Researchers say that it's a nightmare to figure out. In fact, a group of more than 40 academics from a number of disciplines called the Consortium of Functional Glycomics is working with a $34 million grant from the National Institutes of Health to accomplish the task. But even with this hefty federal funding, the scientists admit they won't be able to detail every sugar in the body. That, they say, will likely take many years of difficult research. While mainstream scientists have recognized and are investigating the potential of synthetic glyco-drugs, their efforts may require years to produce results. The increased interest in the role of sugars in human health can expand the market for natural and effective glyconutritional supplements ***today!***

Why Wait?

Fortunately, we don't have to wait for the results of this research before we can begin to give our bodies the help that these sugars offer. The glyconutrient complex offers these necessary sugars in their natural form – not as drugs. The sugars in the glyconutrient complex are harvested from rich plant sources and delivered in easy-to-take glyconutritional supplements. They allow cell-to-cell communications and immune system support to help you stay at your highest level of wellness, which includes the proper functioning of your glands and organs.

As glycomics research starts to increase and gets more attention, it will raise awareness among health professionals that glyconutrition is real and legitimate. They'll soon become more interested and open to the nutritional impact on health, particularly glyconutritional supplements.

Glycomics again, is the total knowledge about sugars(monosaccharides) and how they function. Glycobiology is the study of how sugars support living systems. That means how they affect biological structures and contribute to health in living beings. Most of the researchers in the glycomics field are trying to create synthetic sugar drugs that fight disease. Our research is centered on how these sugars in their natural form impact normal biological processes and the best ways to offer them as supplements. We're not fighting disease; we're sustaining health and wellness – a different approach entirely.

There is no drug for health. If you want health, you must create, protect and sustain it. Glyconutritional supplements (glyconutrient complex, phytonutrient complex, phytosterol complex) are a key ingredient in this process.

"You are what you eat, digest, assimilate, appropriate and eliminate. If you have a problem with any one of these five areas, you will experience nutritional deficiency and cellular contamination, which are the major reasons why people get sick and diseased."

Chapter 15
LETTER TO DOCTORS

The following letter impressed me so much that I had to include it in this book. I heard Dr. Rayburne W. Goen, from Oklahoma, speak three years ago at a health conference in Dallas, Texas. He is a man of great wisdom and has a wonderful sense of humor. His credentials are impeccable. He has the following education and experience: M.D. degree (1939), University of Colorado (Phi Beta Kappa and Alpha Omega Alpha, Honor Medical Society); Lt. Col., Medical Corps, U.S. Army, WWII; Diplomate, American Board of Internal Medicine; Fellow, American College of Physicians (FACP); Fellow, American College of Cardiology (FACC); Clinical Associate Professor of Medicine, University of Oklahoma School of Medicine, Tulsa; past Chairman, Medical Section, St. John Medical Center and for St. Francis Hospital; past Vice President, Medical Staff, St. John Hospital; past President, Medical Staff, St. Francis Hospital; Leader in Medicine Award, Oklahoma State Medical Association.

[Reprinted by permission.]

Dear Doctor:

Thank you for allowing me this opportunity to introduce you to the most monumental discovery in healthcare in the past 100 years, now acknowledged in medical journals and textbooks (1996).

When I first heard about **glyconutrients** four-and-a-half years ago, I called it "hogwash." I declared that anyone who claimed that oral administration of these supplements was of striking benefit to people suffering from a long list of unrelated diseases or ailments was a QUACK . . . in the same class as all the others making such claims, whatever the modality, for relief of a multitude of ailments so blatantly proclaimed and touted in numerous brochures and catalogs in the daily mail. I was already well versed in that kind of hype! I had previously tried on myself, enthusiastically at first, the highly touted glucosamine, chondroitin sulfate, cetyl myristoleate, MSM, SAM-e, blue green algae, alfalfa tea, olive leaf extract, colloidal silver – each with lots of "ink," but not one of them helped me in any way.

I was closed-minded – call it skeptical, dubious, or cynical – as you and the rest of our medical profession would have been, and are. I was, however, receptive enough to read the pertinent medical journals offered to me, and I must admit I was a little jarred at the implications of what I read. I began to look into what turned out to be an overwhelming amount of related literature: Carbohydrate ("glyco") metabolism is suddenly a hot subject – over 20,000 papers in Medline 1996-1998, and a greater number since. All of them are in specialty research journals that we as practicing physicians do not take or read – nor readily understand! The clinical articles published thus far have been mainly retrospective or prospective: case reports of a series of patients with a major disease, and with suspiciously high percentages of positive results. I read many of these articles, but I could not believe they could be documenting something so fundamentally powerful as that a mere food supplement (sugars at that!) could correct a deficiency in our diet so vitally important as to be the mechanism of all cellular communication in our body! The **glyco** of glycoproteins enables every metabolic and biologic function that occurs in that marvel of creation, the human body!

I proposed to try (surreptitiously – "don't tell anybody") glyconutrient supplements for a list of 21 ailments I could identify in myself, rated in severity from 1-10, attributable mostly to "old age" (I was 85 years old at the time). I was not neurotic – just trying to be scientific. None of these completely disabled me, except arthritis of the knees, which required aspiration of fluid and instillation of a cortisone, Depo Medrol, more and more frequently – eventually about every three months for one, then the other knee. Then I would again be functional. I had peripheral neuropathy, which impaired my balance, walking and sleep because of restless legs; a right shoulder rotator cuff tear; low back pain; cervical disc with left C-5 radiculopathy; inflammatory osteoarthritis of hands (I could not shake hands without hurting for the next three days); hypertension (190/105); hypercholesterolemia (320 mg) since in my thirties; nocturia 4-6 times per night; urinary urgency incontinence; prostate cancer; developing cataract left eye, etc. **Within four months I became symptom-free of 20 of these 21 complaints!** I was able to **discontinue all the six prescribed drugs, and all over-the-counter, except one baby aspirin every other day (I had a coronary in 1990 for which I took aspirin). The drugs had been effective to a degree, but all had side effects that were either disagreeable or intolerable.**

That result was not enough to convince me. This had to be some sort of "fluke"!

I resolved I could disprove this "stuff" by persuading a know-it-all patient, who scoffed at the idea of taking supplements like these for his refractory Raynaud's syndrome (cold-sensitive fingers that turned purple and agonizingly painful upon exposure); uncontrolled Type II diabetes with serious adverse effects from insulin and oral anti-diabetes drugs; hypercholesterolemia; and diabetic peripheral neuropathy, worsened by all statin drugs for cholesterol reduction. He was scheduled for replacement surgery of both knees, each of which had been operated on twice for old injuries and loss of cartilage, poorly responding to NSAID drugs and with intolerable side effects. He had stated he was going to discontinue all of the above drugs – he would rather die than live this miserably. I reminded him that dying is an easy out but that he might not die, but be disabled by heart attack, stroke, amputations, blindness or renal failure and dialysis. I managed to induce him to try glyconutritionals for four months, with the assurance they absolutely could not harm him. He reluctantly agreed . . . three weeks later he reported he was free of pain and paresthesias, was having normalized blood sugars on just the one oral anti-diabetes drug he had continued (but that previously had not controlled the high blood sugar); his vision and mental clarity were strikingly improved. He neglected, however, to reorder the supplements and the symptoms all recurred within two weeks. Upon resumption of the supplements, the symptoms again abated. Koch's postulates fulfilled!!

I still was not convinced! I did cautiously offer glyconutrients to several other former patients, including two refractory diabetics with complications, with similar salutary effects. I was nearly convinced after almost a year of results that I could only describe as incredible!

So . . . I gave glyconutritional supplements to Zondra, a patient whom I had "doctored" for 50 years with muscular dystrophy, spinal atrophy type. (Her brother had died at age thirteen with Duchenne type MD.) She was under total care since age three, unable to do anything for herself, had impairment of swallowing, and was on oxygen 24 hours daily. She was able to do some ceramics painting with her right arm supported on a table, for two hours twice a week. Four months after starting glyconutrients she could, for the first time in 50 years, feed herself, brush her teeth, scratch her nose, and is now off oxygen for 3-4 hours daily. She can now swallow well and she can paint 6-8 hours per day, six days a week! She states, "I have so much energy I could do more, but know I should rest some, whether I feel the need or not!"

She has sustained this improvement, and for the first time ever, she has not been treated or hospitalized for respiratory failure or infection in over a year, despite a flu epidemic disabling two of her nurses and her roommate!

Bill, a former surgical technician in the military service, developed Type II diabetes after returning from overseas in the 1980s. When originally diagnosed, his blood sugars were in the 900s and remained uncontrollably high (above 500) for many years, despite multiple injections of regular insulin of up to 200 units daily, plus Ultra-Lente (long-acting) insulin, 120 units daily. He exhibited retinopathy, with bleeding inside both eyes, requiring laser cautery therapy every three months for years, which provided some improvement but could not prevent subsequent recurrences. He developed peripheral neuropathy of both legs and arms with complications of diabetic ulcers on his legs and feet, for which amputation was advised. This he refused, and he experienced considerable muscle deterioration, with claudication (leg cramps) and angina on attempting to walk half a block. He gained weight, up to 330 lbs., with the inactivity. Despite being on multiple anti-hypertension medications, his blood pressure for years averaged 200/115. He developed arthritis, with difficulty doing anything with his hands. After four years, he finally obtained HMO authorization for an electrified scooter, which enabled him to get up and around. In the early 1990s, over a 3-4 month time period, he had a series of strokes and three TIAs. He was diagnosed with sleep apnea, complicated by shortness of breath at rest, necessitating six assorted inhalers, including nasal and tracheo-bronchial steroids. He experienced heart failure with edema of the lower limbs. The strokes left him with some permanent left-sided weakness, migraine headaches, and double vision. For years he has been on a multiplicity of antibiotics – a month without any was considered a good month! His kidneys began to excrete albumin, and his BUN and creatinine elevated as he approached renal failure that would require dialysis. Because of the seriousness of his combined health problems, he "realized this would prove TERMINAL in a short period of time." He became severely depressed because of his condition and by what it was doing to his family. Despite the efforts of 12 doctors and specialists, nothing seemed able to alter the downward trend of his health.

He had "given up ALL HOPE, and was making preparations for his funeral" when he was introduced to glyconutritionals by the minister who would conduct his funeral. After some Internet research, he decided as a last resort to try some – "not expecting anything to happen. After all, nothing else had helped."

Three months later his vision was improving; the ulcers of feet and legs were healed; the pain, swelling, weakness (including the left side stroke weakness), shortness of breath, and angina no longer were a problem. He was off all six inhalers and his arthritis was all but gone. He is able to walk without depending on the scooter or a cane and now drives his car. The migraine has resolved, as has a chronic sinusitis, and he has not needed any more antibiotics. Blood pressure now averages 130/85. The albumin is no longer found in his urine, and the creatinine levels have not increased, indicating stable renal function rather than the previously noted progression. He lost weight, going from 330 lbs. down to 280 lbs. and continues to lose fat and regain muscle mass. The insulin has been reduced to 10-50 units daily of regular, with Ultra-Lente of 60 units each AM and PM. The blood sugars are running 105-125, and the glycohemoglobin (A1c) is now an incredibly low 5.1 (a measure of the biological level of glucose saturation of the red blood cells – very, very good!). He has admittedly not paid enough attention to his diet, and could no doubt reduce his weight and insulin further by following a low-glycemic diet, and now that he is able, he is starting to do more exercise. His severe depression is no more. [After 4+ years of this wellness, he had an accident and fell, injuring his spine. Eventually, meningitis was diagnosed and glyconutrients were stopped during hospitalization and operations. He deteriorated rapidly, with diabetes uncontrolled, paralysis and incontinence of bladder and stools, massive bedsores, ulcerations and bleeding. He is now **near** dying.]

Maxine is a 65-year-old housewife who had breast cancer in 1984, treated with bilateral mastectomy. The cancer recurred in the abdomen and stomach 16 years later, for which she received 6 chemotherapy treatments in 2000. These were very poorly tolerated and did not improve her condition. She developed obstruction of colon, necessitating a colostomy, and blockage in the stomach outlet resulting in abdominal swelling, loss of appetite, and rapid weight loss. She was told there was nothing more to do and hospice was utilized for pain control, with injections of narcotics, and expectation of death within six months. Three months passed, with a downhill course. She and her husband did not give up and sought help from herbs, but without benefit. Glyconutrients were offered to her, and in desperation, she began to take them. Within two weeks she was out of bed, going to church, and a week later she insisted on going to a garage sale! She was then up and around, doing housework and the cooking, enjoying eating, in little pain, and the abdominal swelling had disappeared. Praise God! [Unfortunately, after eight months of comfort and activity, glyconutrients were not available for two weeks, during which time she rapidly declined. When the glyconutrients became again available, she could no longer swallow or retain, and within another week she died. The lesson: if effective, **NEVER, EVER DISCONTINUE THE GLYCONUTRIENTS!**]

The sugars are teamed with other supplements directed toward **protection, regulation, repair, nourishment, and disposal functions**. Glyconutrients are fully documented to be safe, non-toxic, and do not interfere with Rx drugs. We are noting one-third of those taking glyco-supplements show striking improvement; one-third require longer, or larger amounts; and one-third may not respond. Such RESULTS as these, and now many others, I have not seen before in my 64 years as a doctor!! Nothing is ever 100 percent – there must be some other unknown **essentials**, as well as the known: **oxygen, water, and food**: i.e., amino acids, fatty acids, carbohydrates, vitamins, minerals, trace elements. None of those are now likely deficient within our current diet and traditional supplements – except **six of the newly-recognized eight essential sugars**, and possibly the **omega-3 fatty acids**.

The only things that convince most of us doctors are CONSISTENT, SAFE RESULTS. We have all been led down the primrose path with promising new drugs, approved by the FDA, and have seen them withdrawn from the market six months later because of dire effects on the liver, kidneys, bone marrow, GI tract, and/or pregnancy. How many more do we daily prescribe which result in only occasional idiosyncratic lethal effects with approved doses within the acceptable risk-benefit ratio? (But over 106,000 in the year 1997 died in, and 280,000 died outside hospitals from reactions to properly prescribed and taken drugs, as reported in JAMA, July 26, 2000. This is the third leading cause of death in the U.S., outnumbered only by heart attacks and cancer.) It has happened in my practice, as it has in every other doctor's who prescribes for patients. It has been devastating enough to me and you, but how much more so to the patients and their families! For them, it is 100%!

Carbohydrates were always acknowledged to be **just for energy. Not any more!!** Of the 200 known simple saccharides (monosaccharides), there are **eight now recognized to be essential** to all cellular function. They are glucose, galactose, mannose, xylose, fucose (not fructose), N-acetylneuraminic acid (also called sialic acid), N-acetylglucosamine, N-acetylgalactosamine. Six of these eight essential monosaccharides are universally lacking in our diet because of soil depletion, green harvesting, processing, preservatives, and overcooking. Fortunately, our bodies can make the other six from glucose and galactose, **if everything is all right!** Obviously, everything is not all right if the body has a **health problem**, whether from **infections** or **toxins** in our environment: the air we breathe, the food we eat, the water we drink; **stresses** in our lifestyle; **deficiency** of a necessary enzyme, vitamin, co-factor, trace minerals; **free radicals** or a **genetic defect**, in the 15 or more stages, plus much energy to convert one (available) sugar to another!

Currently, the most important one of all these "essentials" is the one that is missing! And "essential" means the body must have it; cannot make it; and without it the body is dysfunctional, sick or dying!

There are some new studies, double-blind, placebo-controlled, with enough numbers to be statistically significant, as we are so used to seeing; but these are years away from being reported. Food supplements, being non-toxic, do not undergo this type of research. Many are not subject to double blinding or placebo control, such as near-terminal cancer cases, genetic disorders with progressive downhill course, and immune dysfunction diseases which are epidemic, overwhelming us over the past 2-3 decades. For these we have no cure – nor even satisfactory or safe relief of the symptoms, with our conventional therapy. Asthma, lupus, hepatitis C, rheumatoid arthritis, osteoarthritis, cancer, ADD-ADHD, fibromyalgia, diabetes Types I and II, chronic fatigue syndrome, multiple sclerosis, AIDS, ulcerative colitis, Crohn's disease, Down syndrome, muscular dystrophy, ALS (Lou Gehrig's disease). These are just a few examples in which administration of glyconutrients has resulted in improvement or remission in each of these conditions (without any harmful side effects!), as documented in reports or publication in peer-reviewed medical journals.

What could possibly be the common denominator of all these? Immune system dysfunction! Why? Something essential is missing!

Glyconutrients are not a treatment, mitigation, or cure for any disease; but if these food supplements are **supplied in the diet, the body can heal itself of virtually anything wrong**! (But not grow a new tooth in an adult if one is pulled, or a new limb if it is amputated. That is not in our DNA! It is, however, in the DNA of sharks which lose a tooth and lobsters which lose a limb!)

These eight monosaccharides are in and on every cell in the body. They are necessary as the glyco of glycoproteins on the surface of every cell, as transmitter or receptor of all the vital reactions between cells: defense, repair, regulation, nutrition, and apoptosis (the programmed death and recycling of all cells). Every cell in the body (600 trillion, give or take one or two) is replaced at different rates, e.g., WBC, 6-7 days; RBCs, 3-4 months; DNA and most internal organs, 6 months; bone, 9 months to years for the femur; brain and spinal cord, 14 months. These monosaccharides are present as a substrate in the endoplasmic reticulum, and as building blocks for the glycosylation occurring in the Golgi apparatus of cells, forming glycoproteins, proteoglycans, glycolipids, glycophospholipids.

This is all under control of the DNA as the blueprint, and mRNA, as the message. The glycoproteins translate the messages and send chemical signals (cytokines) to the appropriate receptors (also glycoproteins), to facilitate the proper action at the cellular level. This is the Universal Code of Life, equivalent to the Microsoft Operating System which runs all computers! This is extremely complicated and has to be not 99.9999% perfect, but 100%, or there is dysfunction, disease, or death! I have studied it intensively, still know so little, but yet enough to be awed and excited by what I have witnessed! Supplying glyconutritionals in the diet has enabled the body to **modulate the immune system**: elevate those elements that are too low, as in cancer and AIDS; and reduce those that are too high, as in autoimmune diseases; or do both, as in most of the immune dysfunctions!! This modulation had been considered impossible – something never before seen in medicine. The **new glyconutrient complex with an antioxidant count that is proven to be by far the most powerful antioxidant of 90 tested in the market is anti-aging, anti-mutation and anti-cancer, by combating free radicals.**

The natural killer (NK) cells, necessary as the first line of defense against infection and cancer, are reduced by 30 percent in even the "normal" population in the past two decades, and are further falling by 3 percent per year. No wonder 150 million of the U.S. population are suffering from some form of acute or chronic disease! These NK cells are restored to normal counts in those receiving glyconutrients.

How? I do not know! But the body knows! Thank God!

Cell-to-cell communication via a "zip code" was the subject for the Nobel Prize in Medicine awarded to Dr. Günter Blobel in 1999. He did not recognize that glycoprotein interactions generated the actual specific chemical messages sent. This mechanism of communication has been demonstrated within the past decade, when use of mass spectrometry and high resolution NMR spectroscopy became available, initially only at Oxford University. In the past few years, eight essential monosaccharides were identified – then the globe scoured for plant sources of the missing monosaccharides. They were identified, isolated, purified, and combined into a powder as a nutraceutical: a pharmaceutical-grade high antioxidant, natural food concentrate.

Dr. Robert K. Murray, senior editor of *Harper's Biochemistry* (Appleton and Lange, 1996), wrote Chapters 56 through 65 on: Glycoproteins; The Eight Essential Monosaccharides; The Extracellular Matrix; Muscle Metabolism; The Immune System; etc.

I now have the 25th edition (2000), and am poring over the awesome biochemical reactions, newly-discovered, in this explosively growing segment of biochemistry: glycoscience, glycobiology, and glycomics!

I will ask you, doctor, if I may, "How did you advertise when you started your medical practice? Newspaper? Radio? TV? Or word-of-mouth from satisfied patients??" I can guess!!! So did I!

Don't knock **word of mouth marketing**! We who are aware of this discovery do not sell products, but educate and introduce the good news to those we love and want to help, who then can order these glyconutrients wholesale from the only company who can supply all of them, shipped directly to their home; to be taken as a **complement to conventional medical care**. We, and they, see benefits more safely, more completely, more consistently, and less expensively, than we have ever seen in our lives before! And **they, in turn, will share** the good news with others who are suffering from the effects of these deficiencies! Better yet, these nutrients enable prevention, wellness and anti-aging!

I am now retired, but I can't deny my love for medicine; nor yet ignore the recent monumental advancements in the science of nutrition – and especially the role of monosaccharides in the formation of glycoproteins, so vital in the function of the cells of our body. At age 89 I am enjoying a new career (yes, mission!) to share with everyone I meet, this epochal nutritional breakthrough and its effect on the immune function. Medicine has advanced beyond the bloodletting, leeches, and maggots treatment of disease to immunizations, wonder drugs, incredible surgery, organ transplants, and DNA/genomes. We have great expectations from the latter, but the promised wondrous cures are yet years away from application, and even the initial genetic modifications are fraught with the same old side-effect complications as other synthetics have exhibited. The body is programmed by God to utilize whatever it needs from our foods, and is not about to change. Stem cell cloning is far from perfect, although it must be invariably perfect, and subject to the same responses to nutritional deficiencies as those we have found so refractory – until the missing glyconutrients are supplied. Glyconutrients are already available here and now, safe and effective, awaiting but the eventual universal recognition by all health professionals! This new nutrition is the keystone of **prevention and wellness**, as our new focus in the practice of medicine, versus the traditional paradigm of treating **sickness symptoms** with Rx drugs.

This new paradigm in medicine did not originate in the traditional "A Drug Cure for Every Disease" concept of pharmacology, nor yet by the nutritionists. This is a disruptive technology, comparable to the displacement of phonograph records with magnetic tape, and this, in turn, by digital CD and DVD, each of which was birthed by a totally unrelated industry. Likewise, was the obsolescence of the watch and clock by the quartz crystal; and the mechanical typewriter by the electric, and this, in turn, by the word processor of the computer, again an upstart industry . . . The new biochemistry: glycobiology, glycoscience, glycomics: glyconutrients!

I couldn't blame you if you thought me a kook – but do please be open-minded, for your own sake, and for that of all your patients. And in so doing, you will honor the aphorism of that wise old doctor, Hippocrates, the Father of Medicine, whose first concern with his patients was, "Primum non nocere." (Above all, do no harm!) And his next was, "Let your food be your medicine, and let your medicine be your food."

What goes around comes around!

Rayburne W. Goen, Sr., M.D.

Arthritis Testimony

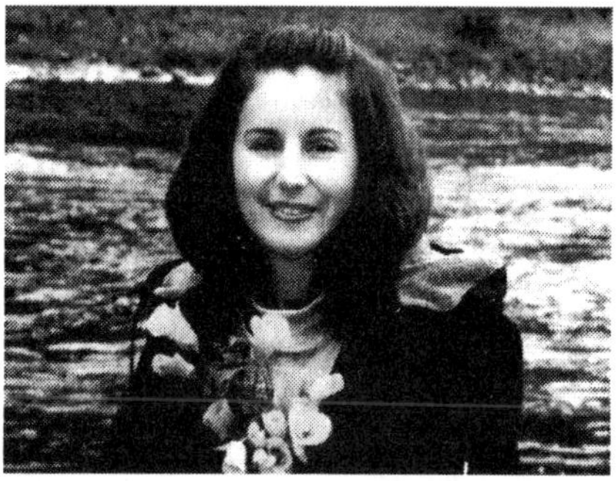

"When I was pregnant with my third child, I started having excruciating pain all the time. I love to walk and run, but I had to stop due to the pain. A doctor said I had arthritis in my pelvic bone; when I heard that, I thought, great – I can't run any more, I can't walk any more. Then, about three years ago I started having a sore throat all the time. So I went to the doctor and he told me that it must be some kind of virus or bacteria that has to be treated. He said we have to up the dosage of the medicine. So I went through this three different times and every single time I was sicker than I was before. Then he told me after the three times of going on medication that I had candida. After that I said I still have pain all over the place. I'm achy, my bones ache, my muscles are extremely tight, I feel like I have the flu all the time. I asked: 'So what else? What is our next step? Do I go to the hospital and get some tests run?' He said, 'No, I can't help you any more.' Then he said he thought that it was all in my mind and that it must be the stress that I have gone through in my life recently.

"So I went on a search for another doctor and I went to this new doctor and he told me that I had fibromyalgia and then I said, 'Okay, so what do I do?' And he said, 'Here are some pamphlets and here is how you can deal with the pain.' I asked, 'Do I have to put up with this the rest of my life?' And he said yes. So I started looking for other alternatives and I tried to change my diet. After six months I still had extreme pain in all the places, except my sore throat had gone away. Changing my diet must have helped this.

"Then I had a cancer patient come to me who had great success with the glyconutritionals, and she shared with me the three products, and a month after I started on the glyconutritionals, I started feeling less back pain. I would have to say three months into it I could definitely see some major changes and by a year and a half I was totally recovered from all my pain and now I am able to run again. I run every morning at 6:00 and I am getting ready to try to run a ten-miler. I feel like I have my life back and it is an answer to my prayers. I have a deep desire to just continue to be there for my children. My husband and I also have three more beautiful kids that are adopted, and so we have six now – four girls and two boys – and I would never have had the strength or the ability to care for them unless I was on these glyconutritionals. They are totally incredible and they are a godsend."

– *Regina*

Chapter 16
FINAL WORDS

Thank you for taking the time to read my book. I want you to know I have no axe to grind, just the truth as I see it and the need to share it. God gave us the law of *cause* and *effect* so that we can take stock of how we are faring. Take advantage of this by studying the *effects* of the way you live. The secret for improving your health and life is in changing the *cause*. Dr. Marcia Smith recently said, "Health is an active pursuit, not a passive result."

Be open-minded but not gullible. Prove all things, hold fast to that which is true, and remember, the bugs only have power over those with weakened immune systems.

What Do the Doctors Think?

Oncologist Glen Hyland, M.D., analyzed H. Foster's evaluation of thousands of cancer cases, many with "spontaneous" remissions. Foster noted they often made major dietary changes. Dr. Hyland noticed a favorable response with four patients that failed all traditional cancer therapy but used nutraceuticals. He noted they had consumed a glyconutrient complex, phytonutrient complex and phytosterol complex. This led Dr. Hyland to evaluate over 100 cases of cancer that had started radiation and/or chemotherapy that improved their diet by adding the above supplements.

Here are Dr. Hyland's conclusions regarding nutraceutical dietary supplements:

1. They do NOT inhibit tumor cell destruction by radiation and chemotherapy.
2. They enhance tumor cell destruction.
3. They protect normal cells from radiation and cytotoxic damage.
4. They induce reductions in malignant tumor masses that were resistant to all treatments.
5. They improve quality of life for patients by reducing toxicity and side effects from radiation and chemotherapy.[30,31]

"The biggest revolutionary change in the war against disease is represented by glyconutrients. If you do not want to become a patient (and therefore a statistic) you need to answer in your own mind and heart if what you are doing for your health is optimal, and if not, what else can you do?" (Michael Schlachter, M.D., is board certified in internal medicine and is a pulmonary disease clinical instructor.)

"I really believe that glyconutrients are something that will become mandatory for overall health, and the reason I have come to this conclusion is because I have spent the past several months doing what I call research on the research. And when I would do searches on glyconutrients, and especially on a lot of different disease processes, I was floored by the number of quality studies that are out there that have shown such benefit and promise in a myriad of diseases ranging from diabetes to arthritis. I believe that glyconutrients are going to become a staple nutritional supplement for all six billion people on the face of this earth within the next three to five years." (Rob Ortmann, M.D., is an immunologist and research scientist.)

A University of California – Irvine study of 196 natural products for toxicity and efficacy found the three multiple-ingredient products containing glyconutrients were non-toxic, caused no cytochrome p450 activity and were effective in all three efficacy assays (NK cell enhancement, antioxidant activity and antiviral effect).[44] I have included in this section Dr. Michael Colgan and Michael Wagner's (BA, LMT, CFT) "No Quick Fix" and "The Seven Principles" articles which beautifully explain what happens when you make health changes and add missing nutrients, taking them consistently.

"When recommending dietary supplements to persons with health deficiencies, one of the most common questions we'll hear is, 'How fast will this stuff work?' If we can help steer people away from the 'quick fix' mentality and, instead, adapt realistic expectations for realizing improved health through nutrition, I believe we've performed a great service. That's because the restoration of genuine optimal health takes time and patience.

"True, there are exceptional cases, especially with exceptional supplements or unique circumstances. Some people begin a dietary supplement regime and realize amazing results. But they are exceptions. And although certain symptoms may have subsided, the body very often has a lot more healing to accomplish over the long term.

"To assist consumers of dietary supplements to 'stay the course' and not quit their program prematurely because they 'weren't seeing anything' we need to educate them. Not only about the supplements in their regime, but about their own body and how nutrition supports the body to effect improvements in overall health.

"To this end, I've found seven principles worth remembering and passing on to those people we wish to see benefit from nutritional supplements and programs.

"**1.** With nutrition, we are not suppressing or manipulating symptoms as with pharmaceuticals. We are not treating conditions as with herbology. We are simply giving the body what it needs to heal itself and rebuild itself anew and this takes time.

"When correcting nutritional deficiencies, while we won't see instant improvements in most cases, we will be promoting true and lasting healing. Pharmaceuticals may sometimes 'work' instantly, yet never address underlying causes and possess unwanted side effects. Contrary to popular thinking, drugs don't heal anything: only the body can do that – when it gets what it needs.

"In Optimum Sports Nutrition, Dr. Michael Colgan explains why patience is the key:

"A principle of nutrition you need to know is physiological dynamics. Unlike drugs, nutrients do not have rapid effects. No quick fix. The business of nutrition is to build a better body. That has to wait on Nature to turn over body cells. A blood cell lasts 60-120 days. In three to four months your whole blood supply is completely replaced. In six months almost all the proteins in your body die and are replaced, even the DNA of your genes. In a year all your bones and even the enamel of your teeth is replaced, constructed entirely out of the nutrients you eat.

"This time course is well illustrated by the course of deficiency diseases. If I remove all the vitamin C from your diet, within four weeks blood vitamin C will drop to zero. But, you will see no symptoms of disease at four weeks. You will have to wait until enough of the healthy cells have been replaced with unhealthy cells. It is another 12 weeks before the symptoms of scurvy start to ravage your body.

"So when you implement an optimum nutrition program, don't expect to see rapid results. In one of our studies at the Colgan Institute, runners were supplemented to try to improve their hemoglobin, hematocrit, and red blood cell count. But after one month of supplementation, there was no improvement at all. After six months, however, all three indices were significantly increased.

"Think of it this way: If you take a neglected houseplant and start feeding and watering it, the leaves may perk up a bit from the improved nutrition. But you have to wait for the old leaves to die off and new leaves to grow before you get a really healthy plant. It is the same with a human body. When you start feeding it better, you have to wait on physiological dynamics of the body to grow new, improved cells in the improved medium. After 18 years in sports nutrition, the shortest program we will give any athlete is 6 months. With patience, nature can do its work and produce its miracles.

"**2.** We are all unique. Individual biochemistries are affected by diet, lifestyle, drug usage, stress, fitness level, genetics, toxins, etc. It's inevitable, therefore, that some persons will respond more rapidly than others to improved nutrition. If you're not experiencing results as fast as you'd like, it could be a factor of any number of things. It might be that the body has priorities other than the one upon which you're focusing. For example, you may want to lose body fat while your body may want to lose a tumor you don't even know you have. Give your body permission to have its own priorities and timetable.

"**3.** Positive health changes can be occurring without your 'feeling something.' Research studies utilizing blood tests, bone density and body fat measurements, etc., confirm this. Improved health begins on the molecular and cellular levels. Later, this may translate into the alleviation or disappearance of specific symptoms and conditions.

"(The already healthy or symptom-free person, especially persons with abundant energy, might take note: Your health benefits from optimal nutrition tend to come in the form of your body's correcting sub-clinical problems – depletions, imbalances and toxic buildups that haven't yet become clinical conditions or 'felt' diseases. In other words, in optimizing and maintaining health, remember 'feeling healthy' really only means 'feeling symptom-free.' Actor Michael Landon was 'feeling great' on national TV: three months later he died of cancer. Virtually everyone can benefit from improved nutrition since, simply by living, toxins accumulate within our bodies, the body wears out and chronic degeneration slowly settles in. Giving the body what it needs to stay healthy can minimize the ravages of modern living and optimize health.)

"**4.** The greatest health benefits of improved nutrition may well come in the later years of life. Regardless of the rate your current health challenge is improving, continued optimum nutrition just makes good sense, since the greatest benefits may be experienced in your senior years. While others are painfully shuffling around nursing homes and tending to medicine schedules, you might be enjoying your summers on the Colorado River and winters in Hawaii. Is this the benefit you want? Learn what your dietary supplements can do for you. Then make an educated choice.

"**5.** If you experience a 'correcting crisis' while on an optimal nutritional program, stay the course – it's working! When your body begins cleaning out toxins, metabolic wastes, parasites, candida die-off and the like, you may experience uncomfortable symptoms. Because you may feel worse before you feel better, it's important to read the articles and books which address this phenomenon so you can better understand this process. The correcting crisis, when understood, is a clear indication that your improved nutrition program is truly working and leading you to improved health.

"**6.** Licensed health care practitioners still make educated guesses as to how long it might take to see a specific health improvement using nutrition. Admittedly an imprecise science, but as a starting point, a holistic medical doctor uses the following formula: For specific health improvements, figure three months, then add one additional month for each year the chronic condition has existed. For example, a chronic condition of 5 years might be expected to see a good improvement within 8 months, provided the body, mind and spirit of the patient gets everything it needs. Experience with nutraceuticals largely indicated the longer the consumption, the greater the benefit.

"**7.** As one very prestigious medical doctor has well stated, dietary supplements ought to carry the warning: 'Not to be taken on an empty spirit.' The human mind and spirit are powerful beyond measure. They can easily override any optimal health plan. They must therefore be in alignment with the healing process. Sometimes the non-physical causes of ill health are poorly understood by the individual dealing with it. If long-term attempts to achieve better health bring minimal or no results, there may be deeper reasons that need exploration.

"Staying mindful of these seven principles of nutrition and healing will hopefully keep all of us out of the trap of quick-fix thinking and help allow us to create the time and patience to achieve true healing and enjoy lasting optimal health."

(Author's comment: Think about this: If we aren't getting the right nutrients for our body or enough of them daily from our diet, wouldn't it be wise to supplement? I had this question addressed to me regarding how long someone had to take supplements: "Do I always have to take supplements?" I said, no, you can stop taking them when you don't need food any more. These supplements are foods and important nutrients that are missing from our food chain and diets – nutrients our bodies need for health and healing . . . True Health Assurance.)

I would like to correct a couple of common misunderstandings. If you have what is euphemistically called "life insurance," I believe the correct name should be death insurance because you only collect when you die, and in reality, it is your beneficiary who gets the money. I am not saying this is bad, it is just that the reference to life insurance is a misnomer. The insurance money is only paid upon one's death.

The other misnomer, "health insurance," I think should be correctly named accident and sickness insurance because you only receive financial remuneration to pay for the hospital, doctors, nurses, tests, drugs and an ambulance, if used. Health insurance is like a free paycheck to illness. But, believe me, when a person gets sick or has an accident, there is no upside; it costs you in more ways than one. In some countries they pay you to stay healthy and the doctors make more money when they don't see their patients because their patients are well. Wellness insurance is designed to help you get well and keep you healthy. A recent article in *USA Today* gave some examples of corporate America's attempt to tackle the problem of climbing insurance rates and employee sickness – dilemmas contributing to lost revenues. Employees at Logan Aluminum in Russelville, Kentucky, receive $200 for filling out a health risk assessment and receive a shared year-end bonus if the company's overall health expenditures went down. Hannaford, a large supermarket chain, offers a $15-a-week discount on health insurance to non-smoking employees. Johnson and Johnson offers its employees a $500 medical insurance discount for those who participate in a wellness program. Look at what Johnson and Johnson is saying about the wellness program: "The annual estimated savings is over $8 million since the inception of a wellness program." I think the optimal health plan consisting of the three natural formulations I have been referring to, plus a low-glycemic diet and regular exercise, is true health insurance that pays you big-time. If you would like to know more about the wellness program for your family or your company, contact the person on page 140 of this book.

Aging should be free from the restrictions of chronic degenerative diseases like cancer, diabetes, arthritis, etc.; our senior years ought to be a time of contribution – *not* a painful crawl toward the grave!

If you dwell on the past, you are fueling failure; learn from the past but live in the now, planning for your healthy future.

A good friend, Franklin H. Ross, Jr., M.D., thinks these glyconutrients are a miracle – and so do I!

I hope this information finds its way into your mind and heart and that you apply it to your life. May God bless and keep you in good health. ◆

REFERENCES AND NOTES

[1] Dr. R. Michael Williams, Professor of Medicine, Northwestern University Medical School, *Enzymes, The Fountain of Life.*

[2] Steve Nugent, N.M.D., Ph.D., "New Perspectives on Nutraceuticals," *The Grapevine* (American Nutraceutical Association), Vol. 2, No. 2.

[3] American Cancer Association and American Heart Association.

[4] C. Wang; R. T. Pivik; R. A. Dykman; "Effects of a Glyconutritional Supplement on Brain Potentials Associated with Language Processing;" April 20, 2002.

[5] C. Wang; R. T. Pivik; R. A. Dykman; "Effects of a Glyconutritional Supplement on Resting Brain Activity," April 20, 2002.

[6] *M.D. News Magazine*, West Coast Edition, Spring 2002.

[7] "Carbohydrates and Glycobiology," *Science* (magazine), March 2001, Vol. 291, No. 5512, pp. 2263-2502.

[8] Bill H. McAnalley, Ph.D., and Eileen Vennum, R.A.C., "Introduction to Glyconutritionals," *GlycoScience & Nutrition* (official publication of *GlycoScience.org: The Nutrition Science Site*), January 1, 2000, Vol. 1, No. 1.

[9] Nobel Prize for Medicine, 1999, Günter Blobel, M.D., Ph.D., see www.glyconutrient.com for link.

[10] R. K. Murray, "Glycoproteins," *Harper's Biochemistry*, eds. R. K. Murray, D. K. Granner, P. A. Mayes and V. W. Rodwell (Appleton and Lange, 1996), pp. 648-666.

[11] T. Gardiner, "Biological Activity of Eight Known Dietary Monosaccharides Required for Glycoprotein Synthesis and Cellular Recognition Processes: Summary," *GlycoScience & Nutrition* (official publication of *GlycoScience.org: The Nutrition Science Site)*, 2000, Vol. 1, No. 13, pp. 1-7.

[12] B. D. Campbell, D. L. Busbee, H. R. McDaniel, "Enhancement of Immune

Function in Rodents Using a Proprietary Complex Mixture of Glyconutritionals," *Proceedings of the Fisher Institute for Medical Research*, 1997, Vol. 1, No. 1, pp. 34-37.

13 T. L. Whiteside and R. B. Herberman, "The Role of Natural Killer Cells in Immune Surveillance of Cancer," *Current Opinions in Immunology*, 1995, Vol. 7, No. 5, pp. 704-710.

14 Stan Lefkowitz, Ph.D., and Doris Lefkowitz, Ph.D., "Comparison of Natural Killer Cell Activation by Selected Nutritional Supplements: An In Vitro Study," *GlycoScience & Nutrition* (official publication of *GlycoScience.org: The Nutrition Science Site*), August 2001, pp. 1-4.

15 M. J. Montvale, "Medical Economics," *2001 Physicians' Desk Reference for Nonprescription Drugs and Dietary Supplements*, pp. 508, 819, 820.

16 "Carbohydrates and Glycobiology," *Science* (magazine), March 2001, Vol. 291, No. 5512, pp. 2263-2502.

17 "Sweet Medicine," *Scientific American*, July 2002.

18 *Acta Anatomica*, the International Journal of Anatomy, Embryology and Cell Biology, 1998, Vol. 161, pp. 1-4.

19 A. M. Mayer, "Historical Changes in the Mineral Content of Fruits and Vegetables," *British Food Journal*, 1997, Vol. 96, No. 6, pp. 207-211.

20 K. M. Fairfield and R. H. Fletcher, "Vitamins for Chronic Disease Prevention in Adults: Scientific Review," *Journal of the American Medical Association*, 2002; Vol. 287, No. 23, pp. 3116-3126.

21 R. H. Fletcher and K. M. Fairfield, "Vitamins for Chronic Disease Prevention in Adults: Clinical Application," *Journal of the American Medical Association*, 2002; Vol. 287, No. 23, pp. 3127-3129.

22 "Dietary Supplement Health and Education Act of 1994 Legislation which Led to the Creation of the Nutraceutical Industry," *Grapevine*, publication of the American Nutraceutical Association, Allen Montgomery, R.Ph., ed., Vol. 1, No. 1.

[23] T. J. Bramley, D. Lerner, M. Sames, "Productivity Losses Related to the Common Cold," *Journal of Occupational Environmental Medicine*, Sept. 2002, pp. 44, 822-829.

[24] "Capitalizing on Carbohydrates," *BIO/TECHNOLOGY*, Vol. 8, 1990.

[25] "Results of Clinical Trials with Antioxidants: A Review," Glycoscience and Nutrition, 2003; 4:3.

[26] National Cancer Institute website: *Science Behind the News; Understanding the Immune System.* http://newscenter.cancer.gov/sciencebehind/immune

[27] Roger Williams, *Nutrition Against Disease*, 1971.

[28] *Journal of the American Medical Association*, July 26, 2000, Vol. 284.

[29] R. S. Mendelsohn, M.D., *Confession of a Medical Heretic*, 1979.

[30] G. Hyland, M.D., *Grapevine*, publication of American Nutraceutical Association, Vol. 1, No. 2.

[31] "A Pilot Survey: Standard Cancer Therapy Combined with Nutraceutical Dietary Supplementation Improves Treatment Responses and Patient Quality of Life," an oral presentation at Comprehensive Cancer Care II: Integrating Complementary and Alternative Therapies, sponsored by Center for Mind-Body Medicine and National Cancer Institute; Hyatt Regency Crystal City, Arlington, VA; June 1999.

[32] M. Jenson, J. Kanaley, L. Roust, et al; "Assessment of Body Composition with Use of Dual-Energy X-Ray Absorptiometry: Evaluation and Comparison with Other Methods," *Mayo Clinic Proceedings*, 1993; Vol. 68, pp. 867-873.

[33] R. H. Nord and R. K. Payne, "Dual-Energy X-Ray Absorptiometry vs. Underwater Weighing: Comparison of Strengths and Weaknesses," *Asia Pacific Journal of Clinical Nutrition*, 1995; Vol. 4, pp. 173-175.

[34] R. N. Pierson, J. Wang, J. C. Thornton, D. P. Kotler, S. B. Heymsfield, D. A. Seber; "Bone Mineral and Body Fat Measurements by Two Absorptiometry Systems: Comparisons with Neutron Activation Analysis," *Calcif Tissue Int*, 1995; Vol. 56, pp. 93-98.

[35] S. J. Pintauro, T. R. Nagy, C. M. Duthie, M. I. Goran; "Cross-Calibration of Fat and Lean Measurements by Dual Energy X-Ray Absorptiometry to Pig Carcass Analysis in the Pediatric Body Weight Range," *American Journal of Clinical Nutrition*, 1996; Vol. 63, pp. 867-873.

[36] Gilbert R. Kaats, "A Nutraceutical Pathway to Optimal Health: A Summary of Clinical Trials," *An Informed Consent Book for Research Subjects*, Health and Medical Research Foundation.

[37] G. R. Kaats, S. C. Keith, H. A. Croft, D. Pullin, W. Squires, J. A. Wise; "Dietary Supplements and a Behavior Modification Plan Improve the Safety and Efficacy of Pharmacotherapy," *Advances in Therapy*, May/June 1998, Vol. 15, No. 3.

[38] G. R. Kaats and S. C. Keith, "Changes in Self-Reported Disease Symptoms during Participation in Program Integrating a Behavior Modification Plan and Glyconutritional Supplements," *Journal of the American Nutraceutical Association*, 1998, in press.

[39] G. R. Kaats, D. Pullin, K. Blum, W. G. Squires, R. A. Woods, "Comparison of Changes in Body Composition with and without Phytochemical Supplements While Following a Behavior Modification Plan," *Journal of Investigative Medicine*, 1997; Vol. 45, p. 291.

[40] G. R. Kaats, D. Pullin, W. Squires, S. C. Keith, L. K. Parker, K. Blum, "Comparisons of Body Composition Changes While Participating in a Behavior Modification Plan with and without Glyconutritional Phytochemical Supplements: A Meta-Analysis," *Journal of the American Medical Association*, 1998, in press.

[41] Walter Willet, Meir Stampfer, primary investigators, "Rebuilding the Food Pyramid," *Scientific American*, January, 2003.

[42] J. Ramberg, "Researchers Drive Another Nail in the Coffin of the USDA Food Guide Pyramid," *GlycoScience.org: The Nutrition Science Site*, 2003.

[43] H. Reg McDaniel, M.D., addressed the U. S. House of Representatives Committee on Government Reform, November 14, 2001; Rayburn House Office Building, 2157 Independence Avenue, Washington, D.C., Hearing Room #2154.

[44] Gurnee, Kira; LeClair, Malena; "An In Vitro Screening Study of 196 Natural Products for Toxicity and Efficacy;" University of California – Irvine, Irvine, California; Winter, 1999; Vol. 2, No. 1, JANA.

“Our Creator made us - body, mind and spirit - we can only experience total health when the physical, mental and spiritual ingredients of health are provided.”

APPENDIX A

PRODUCT INFORMATION

Glyconutrient Complex

This is a new nutrient blend representing a new class of supplements in the nutraceutical category. This glyconutrient complex is probably the most important nutrient for life and health that everyone needs. It provides extraordinary support to the natural defense system. It is the only nutritional supplement that will bring the immune system into a perfect balance, as an immune modulator, raising or lowering an unbalanced system, correcting it to a homeostasis condition and optimal health. This is also a potent blend of antioxidants, a stabilized matrix containing validated ingredients using the gold standard $ORAC_o$ test. The ingredients are water- and fat-soluble antioxidants: quercetin (Vitamin P), Australian bush plum (Bardi plum), mixed tocopherols (Vitamin E), grape seed extract, green tea extract. This blend, along with the co-factors, including the eight special monosaccharides, creates a synergistic, power-packed supplement.

The standardized eight specially selected monosaccharides are: glucose, galactose, fucose, N-acetylglucosamine, mannose, N-acetylgalactosamine, xylose, N-acetylneuraminic acid. One of the leading medical textbooks, *Harper's Biochemistry*, 1996 and subsequent editions, lists these eight monosaccharide sugars in this glyconutrient blend, all of which are essential for healthy human functioning. If we lack any of these eight sugars, the glycoproteins may not be structured properly on cell surface membranes, and therefore, may not communicate correctly or accurately from one cell to the next. Glycoproteins provide the communication link between cells, warning when pathogens are present, sending messages for help when the cell needs it. These monosaccharides are absolutely necessary for the body's creation of glycoforms, the membrane structure on all cell surfaces. The body glycosylates these all-natural plant-based monosaccharides into glycoproteins which are like little antennas on the cell surfaces so that when one antenna touches another antenna on another cell, they can talk to each other. This cell-to-cell communication is vital for any activity of the body. This includes function, structure, and location needs such as "who am I" and "what do I do?" Many doctors and research scientists worldwide are saying, "This is the single most important discovery in the history of medicine." And I'm happy to say it is an all-natural, plant-derived, standardized nutraceutical, not a medical drug.

The product contains no harmful sugars, preservatives, synthetic colorings or chemical stabilizers. It comes in capsules made from vegetable ingredients.

- Strengthens and balances the overall immune system
- Plays a key role in all cellular communication
- Provides extraordinary support for the natural defense mechanisms

Phytonutrient Complex

This is an exclusive standardized complex formulation designed to help maintain optimal health by nutritionally supporting the immune system, with a dozen select vine-ripened, flash freeze-dried fruits and vegetables that are grown in fertile soil, free from chemical fertilizers and toxic pesticides.

With all the pollution, the stress and with the world becoming a microbial super-highway, keeping your immune system in top shape is becoming more and more important these days. Most people do not get enough of the important nutrients found in these specific nine vegetables and three fruits. The nine vegetables are: broccoli, Brussels sprouts, cabbage, carrot, cauliflower, garlic, kale, onion and turnip. The three fruits are: tomato (which is technically a fruit), papaya and pineapple. This phytonutrient complex is designed to help protect against free radicals (bad guys) and carcinogens (very bad guys), enhancing intracellular glutathione activity in support of the immune system and for cell regeneration.

The product contains no harmful sugars, preservatives, synthetic colorings or chemical stabilizers. It comes in capsule and in powder form.

- Builds resistance to disease
- Helps recovery when ill or run-down
- Supports other bodily functions, like cell regeneration
- Supports immune system in many ways

Phytosterol Complex

Every cell in the body is influenced by hormone production or the lack thereof. This standardized phytosterol complex (beta sitosterol) is designed to naturally support your endocrine system. It is a proprietary formula using the dioscorea herb. The wild Mexican yam, which is the best source for dioscorea, is a tuber that can be as large as 40 pounds. In areas of Mexico, where it is a staple instead of beans, rice or potatoes, the women have very few problems with breast and uterine diseases. The plant is a storehouse of phytochemicals called plant sterols not found in our daily diet or in vitamins and minerals. This phytosterol complex is **not** a synthetic hormone, but a safe, natural plant-derived precursor which the body uses to synthesize into the hormones the body needs. Does it cure breast or uterine cancer? No. When ingested, the body transforms the raw, all-natural nutrients, some of the missing factors, so the body can heal and restore itself.

These hormones are necessary for regulating the function of tissues and maintaining homeostasis or a balance in the body. Our standardized phytosterol complex leads the market with one of the highest concentrations of natural plant-based phytoestrogen and steroidal saponins (non-toxic, healthy, natural nutrition) derived from dioscorea villosa, or if you prefer its friendlier name, the wild Mexican yam. Because the naturally occurring levels of ingredients vary greatly from plant to plant, our standardized product ensures that the wild yam used contains optimal levels of the beneficial ingredients.

The product contains no harmful sugars, preservatives, synthetic colorings or chemical stabilizers. The product comes in easy-to-swallow caplet form.

- Supports the conversion of calories to energy
- Helps efficient burning of fat
- Helps support recovery from stress
- Helps support mental alertness
- Promotes sex hormone balance
- Works in harmony with the immune system

For more information, CONTACT:

George Dubouch, Ph.D.
www.Glyconutrient.com
Dubouch@aol.com
1-541-535-9136
9AM to 9PM Pacific Time

These statements have not been evaluated by the Food and Drug Administration. These products are not intended to diagnose, treat, cure or prevent any diseases.

APPENDIX B

PHOTO TESTIMONIALS

"I believe that the greatest crime in the healing arts today is the mindless suppression of symptoms with drugs, especially with our children."

APPENDIX C

MORE TESTIMONIALS

Arthritis Testimony

"Since retiring on full disability with arthritis several years ago, I started looking for nutritional answers to my health problems. When I heard about Dr. Dubouch's 'body, mind and spirit' healing approach, I knew the 11-hour drive to Medford would be worth it. My energy is way up now, my eyes aren't itchy any more, my stomach is much better, and I can lift my arms over my head without arthritic pain for the first time in years."

Lyman H.

Asthma Testimony

"I was diagnosed by medical doctors as having asthma. I had the classic symptoms, including coughing spells during the night and when I would laugh. I experienced almost constant congestion, fatigue and headaches. Drugs and medications had not helped, and in fact had caused undesirable side effects. I heard about Dr. Dubouch's program and his success without using drugs. His program has corrected most of my asthma. I have lots of energy and feel wonderful."

Ramie G.

Brain Damage and Cerebral Palsy Testimony

"Our six-year-old daughter could not walk or speak at age two due to brain damage and cerebral palsy. Rikkea was born nine weeks prematurely. From about the age of one it became very evident that something was not right with her. She was having seizures, constant drooling from the mouth, unable to sit up straight without physical support, chronic constipation, constant upper respiratory and ear infections, crawled everywhere, clenched left fist always held across her chest, constant muscular spasms. She was attending physiotherapy, occupational and speech therapy, regular appointments to see a cranial osteopath, a naturopath, early childhood intervention appointments, a pediatrician; her left leg was always kind of swung out and the list goes on!

"I gave her glyconutrients daily and after a week she got up and walked around the house!! She began speaking clearly in sentences! Very quickly in the weeks and months that followed, Rikkea dramatically improved. Rikkea is now six and attends normal school without a teacher's aid. She has none of the symptoms listed above. She only now has a slight balance problem when walking! Now four years later, she can write, read, skip, run and do things that the average child can accomplish. We are grateful for her cranial osteopath who took the time to tell us about glyconutrients."

Rikkea's Mother

Down Syndrome Testimony

This is a testimonial by a doctor whose daughter was born with Down syndrome. "My wife happens to be a nutritionist and thought the information made sense. So we switched our daughter away from her original program and started her on the glyconutritional products. She has been taking the glyconutrient, the phytonutrient for children and a children's vitamin. She has not been on a single antibiotic this fall or winter. Her body has been able to deal effectively with the colds and influenzas that in the previous years necessitated a lot of antibiotics and decongestants. She also had a follow-up eye exam with her pediatric ophthalmologist. The doctor commented even before seeing her that she would be surprised if our daughter wasn't already going cross-eyed. After the exam the doctor reported to us that not only did she not show any signs of crossed eyes, she was no longer farsighted."

Dr. Tim H.

Kidney Transplant Testimonial

"My father had a kidney transplant ten years ago, at 75! For the first three years, he only ate a phytonutrient supplement. Then, in October of 1996, he started on all the Optimal Health Plan products. Since that time, we have been able to reduce his anti-rejection meds about 75 percent and his kidney function has remained perfect! He is off all Imuran (the doctors feel that is what gave him two different cancers), his Medrol (prednisone) went from 45 mg a week to 4 mg a week and his Neoral reduced from 250 mg a day to 100 mg a day. He is also off his Coumadin, Bactrim (three times a week antibiotic) and I forgot what else. The transplant doctor knows what he's taking and refuses to discuss it with us. His kidney doctor wrote into my dad's personal hospital record that he is on supplements, and, if 'daughter' is not present, nurses must administer as per instructions at bedside!"

Judy

APPENDIX D

MEDICAL DISCLAIMER

Dietary suggestions offered are not meant to substitute for medical diagnosis and physician management. Micronutrients, i.e., nutraceuticals, are not intended to be used to treat, cure or ameliorate a disease or abnormal condition. However, the Dietary Supplement Health and Education Act of 1994 states that optimal nutrition has been shown by scientists to be essential for good health, to prevent disease and to restore health. Thus, normal biochemical synthesis of structure/function compounds by the cells of the body under the control of genes is supported by dietary supplementation. While micronutrients are virtually non-toxic food substances, there can be allergies and hypersensitivity to virtually any substance taken into the body. If an untoward response is experienced, dietary supplements should be discontinued.